. . . [an] *excellent book for students and professionals in forensic psychology, policing and social work.*

Helen Westcott, PhD, The Open University

This book has been written by two people who really understand children. In passing on their knowledge to professionals who engage with children in the interview room, they create opportunities to reduce the trauma of the interview and significantly improve the quality of information obtained.

Writing in a clear and fresh style, the authors have produced a book which is valuable as a point of reference, a day to day tool and as a training aid to develop skills.

Chief Constable A.J. Butler, Gloucestershire Constabulary

This book should be read by all professionals who work with children and could find themselves receiving disclosures of abuse. It is practical, easy to read and full of examples and hints.. It should be a compulsory text for social work students, trainee police officers, law students and professionals already employed in the Criminal Justice and Family Court systems.

A few years ago, a Chief Justice said that it was unnecessary to educate lawyers and judges in the techniques of interviewing children because it was 'just common sense'. The authors show that successful interviewing requires much more than 'common sense'.

Freda Briggs, Professor of Child Development,
University of South Australia

D0260401

A Guide to Interviewing Children

*Essential skills for counsellors, police,
lawyers and social workers*

J. Clare Wilson and Martine Powell

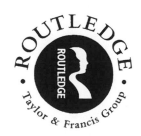

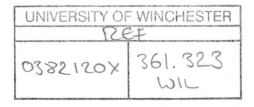
First published in 2001
by Routledge
2 Park Square, Milton Park, Abingdon, Oxon, OX14 4RN

Simultaneously published in the USA and Canada
by Routledge
270 Madison Ave, New York NY 10016

Routledge is an imprint of the Taylor & Francis Group

Transferred to Digital Printing 2006

© 2001 J. Clare Wilson and Martine Powell

Set in 10/11.5 pt Garamond by DOCUPRO, Canberra

British Library Cataloguing in Publication Data
A catalogue record for this book is available from the
British Library

Library of Congress Cataloging in Publication Data
A catalogue record for this book has been requested

ISBN 0-415-25249-0 (hbk)
0-415-25250-4

Publisher's Note
The publisher has gone to great lengths to ensure the quality of this
reprint but points out that some imperfections in the original
may be apparent

Printed and bound by CPI Antony Rowe, Eastbourne

To our parents, John and the late Nancy Wilson,
and Margaret and Lawrie Powell

CONTENTS

*consider? • Are there questions I can prepare in advance?
• Do I need consent from parents to interview a child?
• What do I tell parents when the possibility of abuse is
raised? • What is the best interview environment?
• Should I use toys in an interview? • Should I use a set of
anatomically correct dolls? • When should the interview be
conducted? • What should I do when I first meet the child?
• Why do an initial (pre-interview) assessment? • What are
the ground rules of the interview? • Does telling a child to
say 'I don't know' or 'I don't understand' work? • Who is
the best person(s) to interview a child? • Should a support
person be present during the interview? • What about
videotaping the interview? • Should I get the child's
consent? • How should videos be filed and stored?*

*when working with an interpreter? • How do I encourage
a frightened child to talk? • What should I do when a
child becomes distressed during the interview? • What do I
do when a child refuses to be interviewed? • How do I
tailor an interview to a child who has an intellectual
disability? • What are augmentative and alternative
communication (AAC) methods? • How do I tailor an
interview to a child who has difficulty hearing? • How do
I tailor an interview to a child who has difficulty with
vision? • How do I assess whether a child is responding
with answers just to please me? • How do I assess whether
a child has been coached? • How do I assess ritual abuse?*

TABLES

ACKNOWLEDGMENTS

We are extremely grateful to the many people who have helped with the writing of this book. First, to the children whom we have interviewed or observed being interviewed over the years, and especially those who had the courage to take part in the criminal process. Each child's determination to be heard and understood taught us that the questions are not all-important, listening is. The children's many experiences form the basis of the examples and cases mentioned throughout the book. In order to ensure confidentiality, no source or identifying details are given (except where the transcript has been previously published). Second, to the many police officers, social workers, lawyers and psychologists whom we trained in the interviewing of children. More often than not, it was they who were our teachers. It is the combined wisdom of these two groups that forms the basic philosophy contained in this book.

We also wish to specifically thank Sharon Casey, Merrick Ilett, Teisha Meaney, Lisa McMeeken and David Mellor for their help in the preparation of the manuscript. We are deeply indebted to Chris Boltje and Joanne Bradbury for their comments, insight and ongoing support. We are also extremely grateful to Helen Westcott for reading the first draft and for generally being incredibly supportive and helpful. Our thanks also to Frieda Briggs for believing in us, and to our publisher, Elizabeth Weiss, for her patience and helpful comments. Our deepest thanks to Viviana Cavuoto for her cheerful assistance with the many revisions.

INTRODUCTION

*'First of all,' he said, 'if you can learn a simple trick,
Scout, you'll get along a lot better with all kinds of
folks. You never really understand a person until you
consider things from his point of view—'
'Sir?'
'—until you climb into his skin and walk around in it.'*

Harper Lee (1960), *To Kill a Mockingbird*

Interviewing is about gaining an understanding of another person.
The interviewer asks questions to better appreciate the person she is
interviewing. To climb into that person's skin. It takes immense skill
to climb completely into another's skin. And it takes immense
courage to invite an interviewer in. The foundation of the skill, and
the basis of the courage, is trust. Trust that what is being said will
also be accepted. Not judged. Not applauded. Just accepted.

For a young child, being interviewed requires great courage.
She is likely to have no idea what to expect in the process, or
what the possible outcomes may be. Despite this, she still seeks
acceptance. That she will be listened to. That she will be believed.

To interview a young child takes great knowledge and skill:
knowledge of the language barriers that must be overcome; knowledge of what information needs to be obtained and the skills
needed to access that information; and knowledge that although
the interviewer may want to help, it may not always be possible.
This book cannot give the interviewer the skills needed to
interview a child, only practise can do that. However, it does aim
to give the interviewer the knowledge to inform that practise.

WHO IS THE BOOK FOR?

Primarily, this book was written to help those professionals who
are mandated to interview a child about sexual abuse. A police

officer or social worker or psychologist or psychiatrist may want to assess a child regarding allegations of abuse. A lawyer or judge may want to assess a child's evidence for a trial. The information and techniques outlined here are particularly useful for people in those professions. While the book outlines the interviewing techniques, it does not outline all the legislative requirements regarding the interviewing of a child about sexual abuse. Such requirements (and there are usually a great deal of them) are local to any jurisdiction and country. Every interviewer should be aware of what the local legal requirements are before conducting such an interview with a child.

Child abuse, or other matters concerning a child, may also become an issue for those in professions that normally work with children (e.g. schoolteachers). Further, such professionals may be legally required to report child abuse and may therefore need to discuss such issues with a child—a medic may want to understand how a child has sustained various injuries, or a schoolteacher or counsellor may want to know about bullying or other antisocial behaviour. This book is designed to help them also. While the purpose and goals of these various professions may be very different, the *process* of gaining accurate information from a child is the same.

DOES THE BOOK APPLY ONLY TO SEXUAL ABUSE?

The process of interviewing a child is very similar irrespective of the topic of the interview. While this book focuses on how to interview a child who may have been sexually abused, this is merely one specific illustration of how the interviewing techniques can be used. This example was chosen, not because it requires a particular style of interviewing, but because interviewing a child about such a sensitive topic is the most difficult. Further, interviewers are most often criticized about sexual abuse interviews and such interviews often form the basis of government inquiries into child-protection practice (e.g. the Orkney inquiry).

However, an interviewer may feel that some of the guidelines in this book are more stringent than is necessary—that while an investigation by a police officer into child sexual abuse may require tight guidelines on how to interview a child, it is excessive to apply such guidelines elsewhere. However, the guidelines presented in this book are simple and effective. They should form the basis of all interviews with a child. Casual questions (that a child might not understand) or mild coercion may seem acceptable to an interviewer 'just wanting to explore matters', but they are rarely acceptable to a child.

WHY CAN'T I USE PERSUASION TO ENCOURAGE A CHILD TO TALK?

Some interviewers use mild coercion to encourage a child to talk about sensitive topics (such as abuse). They believe that coercion is unlikely to contaminate the child's report as child allegations of abuse are highly accurate. However, there is scant evidence to either support or deny this assertion. Research can be of little help. It is highly unethical to abuse a large group of children and then interview them over a number of years to see how accurate they are. Although case studies can be evaluated, what actually did happen is usually never known (the same problem exists with records of false allegations—the true rate can only ever be an estimate). What is known is that children's memories for personally stressful events (e.g. medical examinations) can be highly accurate (Goodman, Rudy, Bottoms & Aman 1990) but coercive interviewing techniques may contaminate a young child's report (Ceci & Bruck 1993). The book discusses these coercive techniques to ensure interviewers know when they are using them and how to avoid using them.

WHAT IS THE BOOK SPECIFICALLY ABOUT?

Each chapter of the book represents a step in the interviewing process. Chapter 1 explores how a child views the world and, more importantly, when and where her understanding may differ dramatically from an adult's. Understanding the perspective of a child can be difficult but also enlightening. Without it, the questions asked in an interview may fail and the responses misunderstood. Chapter 2 prepares the interviewer for the interview. To interview a child successfully requires some planning. At the least, a clear purpose for the interview should be well established before the interview. Chapter 3 explains the different interviewing techniques, and gives examples of how best to use these techniques to maximum effect. It also suggests the best structure of the interview, based on international protocols. Chapter 4 gives advice on adapting standard techniques to interview a child from a different cultural background or with some disability. It details the use of interpreters and other interviewing aids. Finally, in Chapter 5, we focus on the aftermath of the interview, particularly on debriefing the child and the interviewer. A full interview transcript is assessed and reviewed to enhance future interviewing skills. Throughout the book, for ease of reading, the gender of 'the child' is kept the same within a chapter and alternated between chapters, except where inappropriate to the context. Also, key references are noted in the text and highlighted in the reference list.

IS THE BOOK RESEARCH-BASED OR PRACTISE-BASED?

The focus of this book is on *how* to interview a child rather than detailing what research has been conducted on interviewing children. There are now some excellent reviews available which summarize the relevant research literature well. For example, on investigative interviewing Poole and Lamb (1998) is highly recommended; Aldridge and Wood (1998) give a good summary of interviewing language; and Sattler (1998) gives a broader and more comprehensive coverage of interviewing children in general. This book, however, is on how to conduct an interview and is designed specifically to answer interviewer questions. We have had to answer many questions both as researchers and as trainers of interviewers, and these questions form the basis for the book. All questions are listed on the contents page so that the book can either be comprehensively read, or 'dipped into' as the need arises. The book would make an excellent companion to a practical training program on interviewing children or can be picked up and used immediately by those professionals 'new to the job' who just need to get started.

HOW DO I USE THE BOOK?

We have designed the book so that it can be used as a quick reference for those with a busy workload. If the interviewer is new to interviewing, however, we recommend that the book be read from beginning to end. It has been kept short, so that this does not take too much of a professional's precious time! The book has also been designed to be interactive. People learn more if they can bring their own experience to learning a new skill. The same principle applies here. There are a number of tasks, some of which can be conducted with a pen and paper and some which require more active involvement. Please do try these tasks. They are discussed in the text as well and suggestions or answers are given in the Appendix, where appropriate.

WHO ARE THE AUTHORS?

Both authors were clinical psychologists before becoming re-searchers. Our research has focused on interviewing techniques and ways to improve the interviewing of children. We have both trained police officers, social workers, lawyers and psychologists in the interviewing of children, working in the United Kingdom, the United States, Australia and New Zealand, where we have also organized practitioner-based conferences on the interviewing of children. We have both made every mistake in the book (and a few that we are not prepared to admit to . . .), and wrote this book as a summary of all we have learned about the interviewing of children.

1

UNDERSTANDING A CHILD'S MIND

To be able to interview a child, one must first have a basic understanding of how a child thinks and communicates. A child's thinking is dependent on a number of factors including memory, conceptual development, emotional development and language formation. To an interviewer the task can seem daunting—to understand all aspects of a child's development in order to conduct an interview with a child. However, the task can be reduced dramatically if the focus is not on all the aspects of child development, but rather on areas of child development that are likely to be important in an interview. What does a child remember and how accurate or reliable are the memories? How does a child understand concepts such as height, weight, age, time, the truth, secrecy and sex? What are common childhood fears? Is a child suggestible? What questions are difficult for a child to understand? The answers to these questions will be age sensitive, that is, as a child matures, cognitive capabilities increase. However, age per se is not always a good predictor of a particular child's abilities. Thinking and communicating will vary from child to child, as each child will have had different learning experiences shaping the rate at which that child develops (Vasta, Haith & Miller 1995). For example, a child who has been grossly neglected is likely to have experienced limited opportunities to encourage development compared to a child of the same age who has received a great deal of positive adult attention.

1

This chapter specifically outlines the different aspects of child development that need to be considered when interviewing a child. However, as rates of development do vary from child to child, the age ranges mentioned should be used as a guide only.

WHAT DOES A CHILD REMEMBER?

> *Box 1.1   Try this*
> Before reading on, write down on a piece of paper everything you can remember about the first ten minutes after you got up this morning. Start from the time you got out of bed and try to remember everything you can. Write down everything, even small things that you don't think are important. Try not to leave anything out.

When you were doing the memory task in Box 1.1, you may have first used knowledge of your home to imagine yourself in your bedroom. Then, using knowledge of what you normally do each morning, you may have prompted yourself to go through the routine: that this morning you got out of bed, had a shower and then had toast for breakfast. You know this because this is what you normally do each morning, and this morning was a normal morning. You do not need to remember all the details of this morning, as it will be similar to every other morning—although you will have some memories specific to this morning. Thus, you reconstructed your morning. Memory is based on reconstruction, that is, no one remembers everything absolutely (Baddeley 1990).

There are three aspects to your description of this morning that are worth discussing further: knowledge, sequencing and prioritizing.

Knowledge

Knowledge is an essential part of remembering. The more you know about something, the easier it is to remember information about it (Thomson & Tulving 1970). For example, a young child may know his favorite storybook by heart, and will get very cross if someone tries to abbreviate the contents. Another child may be able to recall a great deal about 'Thomas the Tank Engine' or

'Bananas in Pyjamas', but at the same time have no idea where he put his other shoe! This is because we tend to seek out information that is important to us. Events or activities that mean a lot to a child will be remembered a great deal more than events that do not interest him at all (e.g. where he left his shoe). In summary, a child's ability to remember an event or activity depends on the amount of knowledge he has—the more meaningful and important the event is to him, the more knowledge he will seek about it, and the better his memory will be.

Box 1.2   Think about this
When a child knows a lot about an event, that child will have a stronger memory about information related to that event. How would that affect a child who knew nothing about sex and was sexually assaulted for the first time compared to a child who had been assaulted a number of times? You will find our suggestions in Appendix 1.

Sequencing

You may have noticed when you were writing down what you did first thing this morning that you automatically ordered the information into a meaningful sequence. The sequence of what you normally do is sometimes referred to as a memory 'script', that is, a list of action details, or routines, of how to do things (Hudson, Fivush & Keubli 1992). Like adults, children have many routine scripts—getting ready for bed, going to school or getting take-away food. In an interview it can be very useful to talk to a child about his routines, as this is usually something he is good at. Further, hearing him talk about his routines gives us a sense of his language and memory ability, and it may also prompt his memory. Anything odd that happens during a routine (e.g. seeing an accident on the way to school) is usually highlighted in the child's memory (Hudson 1988).

Prioritizing

When you described your morning you probably wrote down only the main action details (i.e. what happened). In an interview, we invariably ask about what happened. The main priority is the central details of what happened and these are often remembered by an adult with far greater accuracy than the highly specific or descriptive details (Cole & Loftus 1987). For example, you may have remembered to write down that you had a cup of tea, but may not have reported precisely which cup you chose or from where you took it. However, what is considered to be a 'central' detail to an adult may seem irrelevant to a child. The following excerpt from a court case demonstrates how a child may see some aspects of the abuse as more important (and, therefore, more central) than the main offence:

> Lawyer: What did he do with his penis?
> Ten-year-old boy: I don't know, he was on top of me and he was real heavy, I couldn't breathe.
> Lawyer: So you have no idea what he was doing with his penis?
> Ten-year-old boy: I just remember I couldn't breathe, I really couldn't breathe.

In this case, the interviewer was attempting to establish the exact nature of the offence, which he saw as the central aspect of the abuse. However, the child had thought he was going to die from suffocation and was more concerned to tell the court about that.

While obtaining a good account of the main details may be important in an interview, descriptive information such as where the event took place, where other people were and what the person looked like may also be needed. In our everyday conversations we hardly ever give descriptive details, so a child often thinks that such information is irrelevant. In the interview situation, if specific descriptive details are requested without explanation, a child may feel that the interviewer does not believe him and is trying to catch him out. It is, therefore, a good idea to explain to a child that as you were not there you need to get a picture of what happened—that hearing about things in detail will help you clearly understand what happened.

As a general rule, the younger the child, the less knowledge and routine information he will have and, subsequently, the less detail he will recall (Nelson & Gruendel 1986). Yet, a three-year-old can still accurately report some events that happened a year earlier (Hudson & Fivush 1991). Further, young children can be better at describing routine information than other action details, so it can be useful to start an interview with a preschooler by asking him about the routines in his day.

4

HOW ACCURATE AND RELIABLE ARE A CHILD'S MEMORIES?

Memory is complex and is affected by many factors operating at the time of the event, for example, the time of day, level of stress experienced by the child, where the child's attention was focused, or the time delay between the abusive incident and the interview. In some circumstances, memory can be highly detailed, accurate and persistent. In one study reported by Pipe et al. (1999), five- to ten-year-old children were able to remember and accurately report information (including new information that they had not reported at earlier interviews) two years after an event. In other circumstances, however, memories can be rapidly forgotten or distorted. Probably what many people mean when they ask this question is, 'Can children provide forensically relevant and accurate information and how young can they do so?' The answer to this is more clear-cut. A three-year-old child can provide detailed and accurate information, although his ability to remember and express information will increase with age. Further, personally significant information is remembered better than other types of information (Goodman et al. 1990).

The main problem with the reliability of a child's report is not his memory per se, but the way the interviewer conducts the interview. Even though a young child's memories may be more vulnerable to suggestions from the interviewer than an older child's memories, the onus is always on the interviewer to ask questions that maximize the accuracy of the child's report (see later section in this chapter on suggestibility and Chapter 3 on how to do this).

WHEN DOES A CHILD UNDERSTAND MEASUREMENTS?

Initially a child's thinking is very concrete and relates to information about what can be seen, heard, smelt, touched and tasted. In time, a child comes to use more abstract information, including mathematical and hypothetical concepts. However, it is not until the teenage years that a child totally masters abstract concepts (Seifert & Hoffnung 1997). As measurements are abstract concepts, a young child will not easily understand them, as this transcript shows:

> Interviewer: How old is Malcolm?
> Five-year-old child: He's very, very old.
> Interviewer: How old in years?
> Five-year-old child: Twenty.

In this example, the highest number the child knew was twenty, so he thought that was extremely old.

A child will sometimes use concrete objects to understand abstract ones. For example, up until the age of eight, a child may use a person's height to guess his age. Thus, a small elderly lady may be described as being younger than a tall teenage boy (Wood 1981). Asking a child to estimate the height and weight of another person (e.g. in centimeters or feet, pounds or kilos) is asking him to use units of measurement that he may not know anything about. The phrase 'five foot tall' is only meaningful if you know how large one foot is, can count to five, and can imagine what five feet put together might look like. If measurements are needed, ask the child if the person is about as tall (or as big) as someone else the child knows well. A child will normally find it easier if he can use someone else for comparison.

> *Box 1.3   Try this*
> Next time you are in a cafe, supermarket or other public place, try to estimate the age, height and weight of the people around you. How accurate do you think you would be? Would you be happy for them to know your estimates? Now, imagine how much harder the task would be if you were trying to estimate the age, height and weight of these same people from memory.

HOW DOES A CHILD UNDERSTAND TIME?

A child does not naturally understand time in a discrete, measured way according to the clock. We must all be taught to do this. Rather, a child locates the time of day or year using qualitative rather than quantitative terms—describing where he was at the time, or what other things were happening around that time (Friedman 1991). When a child tries to describe the length of an event, he may instead report the intensity of the experience. For example, when asked about a violent domestic dispute that lasted ten minutes, an eight-year-old child said: 'It felt like forever, it just went on and on.' Some people misinterpret this as sheer exaggeration or inconsistency on the child's part when actually

6

the child is using a different definition of time. Indeed, most of us do experience time this way—a good day appears to fly by and a bad day drags on. By the ages of eight or nine years, however, a child comes to understand clock time, usually as part of his schooling or because he owns and can use a watch. As one eight-year-old girl replied when asked what questions were difficult to answer in court, 'They were asking me about times and last year I couldn't tell the time. My mum got me a watch at Christmas and now I can tell the time. But I didn't know the times they were asking me about' (as cited by Murray 1995).

General approximations of the length of time make more useful questions than exact time quantities. For example, instead of asking 'Exactly how long were you there for?', you could try 'Were you there for a whole day, half a day or less than half a day?' Questions such as 'How long ago?' will be difficult for a child to answer until late childhood. When trying to pinpoint the time of an event in the past, a child should be encouraged to use events that are meaningful to him, for example, the class he was in, whether it was school holidays, what television shows or social events were on at the time. Perhaps the child's parent or teacher can indicate significant events in the child's routine or yearly calendar that may be useful to ask about, for example, Christmas, Chinese New Year, birthday, Passover etc. For example, 'Was it before or after Christmas/Easter/your birthday?', 'Was it a school day or a weekend?', 'Were you in Mrs Brown's class or a different class?', 'Were you living at your new house or your old house?'

The last three examples above are likely to be more effective than the first example because they rely solely on contextual cues rather than temporal terms such as 'before' and 'after'. These terms are not always fully understood until seven or eight years of age (Walker 1994). Thus, the terms 'before' and 'after' should only be used if the child understands them. You can find out a child's understanding of the term 'before' by asking him to count to five and then asking him which number comes before the number three. If the child cannot do this, ask, 'When counting, which comes first, two or three?' Sometimes a child knows the term 'first' prior to learning the term 'before' (Walker 1994).

A child between four and five years of age can usually localize an event by time of day (morning, afternoon, bedtime) while an older child (six to eight years of age) can use longer time scales such as days of the week and seasons (Friedman, 1991). If forced choice options are offered to a child—'Was it morning, afternoon, or night?'—the child should be asked to explain his response—

'How do you know?' or 'What makes you say that?' This helps the interviewer determine whether the child has merely selected a response to please the interviewer.

WHAT DOES A CHILD KNOW ABOUT SEX?

Research on children's understanding of sex and sexuality has been limited for ethical reasons. (For an excellent review of the literature see Volbert & van der Zanden 1996.) Nevertheless, three aspects are clear. First, there are stages of development relating to when a child seeks out information about sex. In general terms, a child between the ages of two and three years tends to identify girls as girls and boys as boys (noting some genital differences) although he can generally label male parts better than female parts and he shows little or no knowledge of adult sexual behavior. A child between the ages of four and five years may demonstrate some knowledge of pregnancy (intra-uterine growth). An older child may describe mainly non-sexual roles in procreation, but knowledge of adult sex rapidly increases as puberty approaches. Around 50 per cent of children who are ten to twelve years of age are aware of sexual touching, masturbation and intercourse (Wurtele & Miller-Perrin 1992). However, an older child may still be unsure about certain sexual concepts, for example, 'intercourse', 'seminal emission' or 'ejaculation' (Volbert & van der Zanden 1996), as are some adults.

Second, as mentioned earlier, a child's conceptual development depends on his experiences. This is also the case when talking about sex. A child's understanding of sex is not exclusively related to age, but depends on what information and experiences he has had (e.g. a child will typically use his parents' or peers' labels for body parts or sexual acts). These terms can vary markedly between regions and even families.

Third, experience per se doesn't necessarily dictate how much sexual-related information the child will *report* in the interview. The likelihood that a child will disclose sensitive information about sex will depend on other factors as well. A child (especially an older child) may be very embarrassed about talking to an adult stranger about sex and so may omit information that he knows or may use slang phrases to imply he knows 'everything' when he does not. To check out the child's understanding of the slang phrase, explain to him that you are unsure what that phrase means and you would like him to explain it. Be careful not to appear like you are testing the child as this may make the child feel stupid or defensive.

Sex is a sensitive topic and an interviewer as well as a child can run into difficulty. For example, the following was a lawyer's attempt to make an ambiguous phrase ('feel' as in touch, as opposed to 'feel' as an emotion) more concrete for an eight-year-old child.

> Lawyer: What did the penis feel like?
> Child: Yucky.
> Lawyer: No, I mean what did the penis *feel* like?
> Child: Horrible.
> Lawyer: No, I mean did it feel like a cold sausage stuck up your bum?
> Child: I've never had a cold sausage stuck up my bum.

Needless to say, it is a good idea to avoid using the term 'feel' when you want to ask a child about touch, especially for abusive events. A child may mistakenly suppose the word refers to his emotional reaction. It would have been more appropriate for the lawyer to ask, 'Was the penis hard or soft?' and then, 'How did you know that?' The second question needs to be asked to make sure that the child isn't guessing the answer to the first question. A preschooler, however, may have no idea how he 'knows' something so you may need to ask for a description of it first. Further, touch may be a more complicated issue for a child who is disabled or chronically sick, because many people could be in physical contact with them. Discussing this with the child's carer before the interview will clarify how best to talk to such a child about touch.

Other problems that interviewers have when talking about sexual abuse usually relate to pinpointing whether the child was touched 'in' or 'outside' the body. For example, a child reports: 'Joe touched my front bottom'. This does not indicate whether Joe touched the child over or under her clothes or whether the child was wearing any clothes at all. To clarify this, interviewers often directly question the child further—'Did you have any clothes on?' or 'Did he put his hand inside you?' However, these direct questions do not establish whether the child understands the terms being used. A child may not know the feeling of having something 'inside' her body. Often they know the word 'inside' only in the limited context of 'Come inside, it's raining!' (Walker 1994). Try to obtain a more detailed answer from the child by gently asking, 'How do you know that he touched you inside?' or 'Tell me more about what Joe was doing.' If the child simply reports that it hurt her or that she could feel it, encourage her to indicate where the sensation occurred. Next, establish the child's understanding of the terms that you both use. For a preschool child, a demonstration may be useful. With the aid of building blocks, ask the child to put a doll 'on top of' the house, 'inside' the house, 'outside' the house, etc.

> **Box 1.4   Try this**
> A child is not always given the appropriate words to describe the genital area and may use words like 'fairy' for vulva, 'teapot' for penis or, more commonly, 'front bottom' and 'back bottom'. Take a few minutes to write down how you would find out what phrases the child uses. What would you ask the child? Would you use drawings or ask the child to point to his/her own body? Why? How would you ask about sexual acts? Have a go at phrasing some questions. You will find our suggestions in Appendix 1.

WHAT IS A CHILD NORMALLY FEARFUL AND ANXIOUS ABOUT?

When interviewing a child, it is useful to know his fears and anxieties. Table 1.1 outlines common sources of fear and anxiety among children and adolescents.

It is worth noting that as the child's world expands, so do the types of fears. For example, a one-year-old is very unlikely to be afraid of witches or ghosts as he does not know what witches are, let alone whether he should be scared of them or not.

As Table 1.1 indicates, it is considered developmentally appropriate for a child aged between two and four years to respond to strangers or new adults with fear, and this can apply to a caregiver that has undergone a sudden change in appearance. For example, if an absent father shaves off his beard, cuts his hair and loses weight, he may not be recognizable to his three-year-old child the next time he comes to visit. As a result the child may become frightened. Likewise, a six-year-old's obsession with witches should not be automatically taken to indicate he is involved in a cult. The source of the child's concerns would need to be carefully investigated. Did it come from a computer game, movie or television program? Being aware of a child's favorite stories, games, and television programs can help in an interview, especially as a child's

Table 1.1 Common sources of fear and anxiety among children and adolescents

Age	Examples of a source of fear and anxiety
0–12 mths	Loud noises (e.g. thunder), certain smells, hunger, spiders, snakes (it is thought that most mammals are born with a fear of spiders and snakes), sudden unexpected and looming objects
1 yr	Separation from parent, falling into a toilet, being injured, strangers
2 yrs	Multitude of sources, including loud noises, animals, darkness, separation from parent, changes in personal environment, strange peers, parents' moods
3–5 yrs	Masks, darkness, animals, separation from parent, noises, bodily injury
6–8 yrs	Supernatural beings, bodily injury, thunder, darkness, sleeping or staying alone, media events (e.g. news report on child kidnapping, nuclear holocaust)
9–12 yrs	Tests in school, school performance, bodily injury, physical appearance, death, parental divorce
Teens	Social performance, sexuality, personal relationships, parental divorce

(Adapted from Harnett Sheehan, Sheehan & Shaw 1988.)

knowledge from these sources can in some cases be mistaken for direct experience. For example, a four-year-old child in one case was terrified that a 'big man' was going to hurt him. The child had seen him on the television stare directly at him and say, 'I'm coming to get you'. It turned out he was an actor in an advertisement.

WHEN IS A CHILD SUGGESTIBLE?

Suggestibility refers to the degree to which a child's reporting of events can be influenced by a range of social as well as psychological factors operating before or after the event being reported (Ceci & Bruck 1993). This definition allows for the many situations where an interviewer can influence what a child says using leading questions or letting the child know the interviewer's expectations and stereotypes. These interviewing techniques may alter a child's reports, irrespective of what the child actually remembers. This is because a desire to please the interviewer may outweigh a desire to be accurately heard. Table 1.2 briefly lists the main factors that are currently known to affect a child's suggestibility and provides a brief explanation of their impact. Note that the greater the number of these factors present in an interview, the greater the possibility that the child's report will be affected.

Table 1.2 Factors known to affect children's suggestibility

Factor	Qualification
Age	Preschoolers are more suggestible than older children and adults because of a smaller knowledge base, limited language and source monitoring (where and how something learned) skills, and an increased desire to please an authoritative interviewer.
Delay between event and interview	The likelihood of reporting misinformation increases over time as actual details of an event are forgotten.
Status of the interviewer	Older, more knowledgable and authoritative interviewers are able to sway children more than low status adults or peers.
Interviewer bias	Sometimes interviewers inadvertently attempt to shape the child's report to accord with their own preconceptions.
Repeated interviewing	Children in subsequent interviews can reproduce false information suggested previously. In fact, simply asking children to repeatedly think about or imagine a fictional event can lead young children to agree that the event happened. If an interviewer frequently repeats a question within an interview, the child may think that the first answer was wrong and she should change it.
Stereotyping	Communicating a negative stereotype of a person or an event can lead children to provide responses consistent with that stereotype; e.g. merely implying someone is bad can result in a child reporting that the person had lied or cheated when he had not done these things.
Peer pressure	A child may report false information to make it consistent with that of a peer.
Reinforcing certain answers	Answers may be shaped through (unintentional) bribes (e.g. 'Just tell me what happened, then we'll stop') and rewards (e.g. 'You're such a good girl for saying this!').
Type of question	Specific questions (e.g. 'What color was his hat?') have greater potential for error than general questions (e.g. 'What did he look like?'). This is because the information in the specific question may not be accurate (e.g. it assumes that the man has a hat and the child knows the color of it). Leading questions (e.g. 'He was wearing a hat, wasn't he?') tell the child what type of information is wanted. The interviewer's tone, manner or phrasing can also suggest that a particular response is desired.

Table 1.2 (cont)

Factor	Qualification
Visualization and socio-dramatic play	False disclosures of child sexual abuse can sometimes occur in response to techniques involving fantasy, imagery, visualization and re-enactment during play. Repeated visualization of events can lead to errors in monitoring the source of the events (i.e. confusing an imagined event for something that really happened).

(See Ceci, Powell & Crossman 1999 for more information on these points.)

While children are more suggestible than adults, suggestibility is a matter of degree only. No age group (not even adults) is immune to suggestion and there are large differences in the extent to which an individual child may resist suggestions (Quas, Qin, Schaaf & Goodman 1997). Further, a child may be highly suggestible in some circumstances, while in other situations he is not. When a child is interviewed appropriately, even a young child can give very accurate accounts. Therefore, the information contained in Table 1.2 should not be used to undermine the credibility of a child, but to highlight to interviewers the techniques that are best avoided when interviewing children.

As a final note, some interviewers may confuse the terms 'suggestibility' and 'False Memory Syndrome' (See Read & Lindsay 1997 for a review). These are very different concepts. False Memory Syndrome refers to a cultivated memory that may have no basis in what has actually happened to a person. As discussed above, being suggestible (for example, saying yes to an interviewer's leading question) may reflect a false belief that suggested information is true, or it may be the result of confusion in the questioning or a desire to go along with what the interviewer is saying. (For further discussion on false memories, recovered memories and trauma see Read and Lindsay 1997.)

Box 1.5 Think about this
In a custody dispute, suppose a parent wanted to convince a child that the other parent had abused that child so that the first parent would get sole custody. How might the parent go about this? How difficult would it be? Could a child make up such a claim by herself? You will find our suggestions in Appendix 1.

WHEN CAN A CHILD BE TRUSTED TO TELL THE TRUTH?

Contrary to popular belief, the younger the child is, the more likely he is to tell the truth. This is because a very young child has yet to learn how to lie. By the age of two, young children can demonstrate deception (Chandler, Fritz & Hala 1989). However, it is around the age of four to six years that a child is able to detect and convincingly tell lies. A child in this age range may consider a lie to be any untrue statement regardless of the intention to deceive (e.g. 'I'm four not five, you are a liar!') and that lying is morally wrong (Peterson 1991). A more adult-like understanding of lying begins to develop around the age of eight when a child will start to understand that lying involves an intention to deceive and how to apply different deceptive behaviors to different situations (e.g. Pipe & Wilson 1994). For example, a child may tell his mother that he did his homework at his father's house over the weekend, and tell his father that the homework was done at his mother's house before coming over. The child understands his parents are unlikely to discuss this issue and therefore he is unlikely to be caught out.

Most adults think that they can tell when a child is lying, but the truth is that adults are very poor judges of lies. There is little we can do during an interview that can accurately detect a lie told by a child (Bussey 1992). We tend to think that the guilty look gives a child away. However, often the 'guilty' look is not the result of guilt at all but of being nervous. When a child is nervous, often he will not maintain eye contact, and he will speak hesitantly and fidget (that is, appear guilty).

HOW DO I ASK A CHILD ABOUT THE COMPETENCY TEST?

The competency test is an assessment of whether a child under-stands the duty to tell the truth, and is usually conducted for legal purposes. If you are interviewing children about abusive incidents for a criminal prosecution you may need to conduct a competency test. It is a good idea to check that a competency test is still required in your area and, if so, what type. Does the competency test involve the child understanding the need to tell the truth? Does it require the child to demonstrate an understanding of deception? Or does it merely involve the child demonstrating the ability to accurately and reliably answer questions? (See Walker 1994 for further discussion.)

If you need to test that a child knows the difference between a truth and a lie, it is better to first concentrate on what the child believes a lie is. Try not to ask a child, 'Tell me the difference between the truth and a lie.', as he will often reply, 'The truth is when you . . . um . . . tell the truth and a lie is when you lie'. The following example illustrates how definitions such as this can be avoided:

> Interviewer: I want to talk about what it means to tell the truth or to tell a lie. What do you think a lie is?
> Child: Like if my brother says he took my truck but he didn't.
> Interviewer: I see, so a lie is something that didn't happen.
> Child: Yeah.

A child will often refer to a lie as something that 'didn't happen', but if he doesn't (as in this example), it is useful to refer to the phrase yourself. If the child has not given a good description of a lie you will need to get him to respond to a practical example. In this case, color references (e.g. 'If I said you were wearing a red sweater, would that be the truth or a lie?') should be avoided as the child may be color-blind, and a very young child may not know his colors. Instead, actions or situations that the child has participated in are less ambiguous. For example, if you picked up the child in a car and drove him to the interview, you could ask, 'If I said that we caught a bus to get here today, is that a lie or is that what really happened?' If the child says a lie, you could then ask, 'Why is that a lie?'

Once the child has defined a lie (i.e. something that didn't happen), then his understanding of the importance of telling the truth (i.e. something that really did happen) can be assessed. This can be in the form of a statement, that is, 'It is very important that we both talk about things that have really happened'. It can also be in the form of a question that requires the child to respond, for example, 'Do you think it is important to only tell me what really happened?', or 'Is it a good or bad thing to tell a lie?' However, the latter questions are not particularly helpful as they merely require yes/no answers (see Chapter 3).

HOW DOES A CHILD UNDERSTAND SECRETS?

Normally, a child will be able to lie before he can keep a secret, as a child needs to know how to lie to conceal a secret. Thus, a two- to three-year-old child may have difficulty keeping secrets. It can be very obvious when a young child begins to keep secrets.

15

The child is likely to get very excited and will be desperate to tell someone that he knows something that others don't. In doing so, he invariably tells the secret (e.g. a sibling's or parent's birthday present). A child between the ages of four and six years can keep secrets well. At this age, the child appears to be 'rule bound' and tends to think a secret is something that you tell 'no one'. He understands that he knows something others don't know and that the person who told him not to tell may be offended or angry if he does so (Wilson & Pipe 1995). A child between the ages of seven and nine years is beginning to learn when it is okay to tell a secret and when it is not, that is, whether he will be punished. From the age of nine years, a child becomes similar to adults in his understanding of who he can tell and when it is appropriate to tell. This will depend on the consequences of telling and his own concept of justice.

The most successful strategy in getting a child to tell a secret is to give him time to get to know and trust you. Secrecy is about trust and so is the sharing of secrets.

> **Box 1.6   Think about this**
> A five-year-old child may think it is very bad to lie and may also report that a secret is something that you don't tell anyone. Yet in order to keep a secret, she must lie. How do you think a five-year-old would feel about telling a secret or lying to keep it? For the child, which would be worse? You will find our suggestions in Appendix 1.

DOES A YOUNG CHILD'S MENTAL ABILITY MAKE HIM VULNERABLE TO ABUSE?

By seven or eight years of age a child's thinking becomes less concrete and more abstract (Flavell 1985). Until this age, a child may find it difficult to reason by implication (e.g. Joe is drunk; Joe is violent when drunk; therefore, Joe may get violent). A child may also have difficulty remembering where and how he learned something (this is called 'source monitoring') (Roberts 2000). Without the ability to connect ideas and to understand the consequences of behavior, a child can find it difficult to understand that someone's behavior is intentional. A young child may have

16

no sense of what sexual exploitation is and may believe that sex is special, fun or normal (Kuehnle 1996). Further, there may be no negative symptoms arising from the abuse and so the child may think there is nothing to disclose. This may be especially problematic for children who have limited abilities (e.g. learning difficulties—see Chapter 4 for further discussion on learning disabilities).

A child's concrete thinking may also make it difficult for him to see the illogical nature of his own and other's stories. For example, he may genuinely believe an adult's claims that the adult has special powers (e.g. that he will automatically know when the child has told others). These factors can reduce the likelihood that the child will disclose anything.

The limits to a child's understanding also have implications for false allegations. A lack of understanding about the full consequences of telling may explain why false allegations for the purpose of revenge or scapegoating rarely emerge until eleven or twelve years of age (Kuehnle 1996).

WHAT DO I NEED TO KNOW ABOUT A CHILD'S LANGUAGE ABILITY?

A child is initially very literal in his understanding of words. This is illustrated in the following example of a five-year-old child being cross-examined in court (as cited in Berliner & Barbieri 1984):

> Lawyer: You said you put your mouth on his penis?
> Child: No.
> Lawyer: You didn't say that?
> Child: No.
> Lawyer: Did you ever put your mouth on his penis?
> Child: No.
> Lawyer: Well, why did you tell your mother that your dad put his penis in your mouth?
> Child: My brother told me to.
>
> (Lawyer for the prosecution tries to clarify the child's comments.)
>
> Lawyer: Jennie, you said that you didn't put your mouth on Daddy's penis. Is that right?
> Child: Yes.
> Lawyer: Did Daddy put his penis in your mouth?
> Child: Yes.

17

Lawyer: Did you tell your mom?
Child: Yes.
Lawyer: What made you decide to tell?
Child: My brother and I talked about it, and he said I better tell or Dad would just keep doing it.

The above example shows how a child can appear to be contradicting herself when she is actually taking the interviewer's question more literally than he intended.

A child may also only use or understand a word in a certain context (as indicated earlier in this chapter). This is because his language skills are learned in the environment in which he lives and, therefore, his understanding of words may be limited to specific contexts. For example, a child may understand what his mother means when she says, 'Do not run in and out of the house!' However, he may not understand the terms 'in' and 'out' when used in other phrases—'Did he have his shirt out or in?' or 'Did she ever have it out with you?' A child will gradually develop a broader definition of words and phrases as he hears them in a greater variety of ways and places. Because every child's experiences and language skills are unique, a child will acquire broad definitions at different times (Walker & Warren 1995).

Once a child starts school he usually learns to use language less idiosyncratically. This is because his peers and teachers will moderate his developing skills. Thus, from school age, a child may talk more like an adult but that doesn't mean he understands language in the same way. Many complex language rules are still to be learned as well as the various meanings each word can have. For example, it is not until a child reaches about the age of twelve that he will begin to detect ambiguity in sentence structure, for example, 'What did it feel like?' referring to touch or emotions (Walker 1994).

To begin with, a young child will have a limited vocabulary and tends to overgeneralize (e.g. any animal with four legs is called a 'dog'.) On the other hand, some words are under-generalized as in 'Did Joe touch you?', 'No, he pinched me'.

A five- to six-year-old child will have a more extensive vocabulary than a toddler but will tend to overgeneralize grammatical constructions, for example, adding 'ed' to the end of verbs to create past tense as in 'I runned away as fast as I could'. Confusion may also arise if the child mistakes an unfamiliar word for a similar sounding word with a different meaning. For example, a five-year-old girl reported to the court that her father had told her that he wanted to show her his spunk (slang for sperm) and when asked what that was, she described a black and white animal that smells (a skunk).

WHAT QUESTIONS ARE DIFFICULT FOR A CHILD TO ANSWER?

There are three aspects to questions that children have difficulty coping with: the type of information asked for in the question (i.e. the concepts asked about); the way that information is asked for (i.e. the grammar used); and the form the question takes (i.e. yes/no or one of the so-called wh-questions). Each of these factors will be discussed in turn.

Concepts

As we have seen, a child's level of conceptual development and life experience will predict what concepts he can and cannot understand. There are many concepts that a young child might have difficulty with. Some have already been discussed (measurements, sex and lies). Other difficult concepts include body parts ('What do you call this?', the interviewer points to the abdominal area, the child replies, 'A shirt'); locations ('Where do you live?', 'At my house'); and taking another's perspective ('Did he see you?', 'Yes', because *she* saw him—she may have no idea if he saw *her*).

Grammar/sentence structure

Sentence structure is an important factor to consider. Interviewers sometimes assume that just because the child knows all the individual words in a sentence, he will be able to understand the whole sentence (Saywitz 1995). Note the way the lawyer in the following excerpt questioned a ten-year-old child about being asked to keep information secret: 'And did your mother ever say to you that if somebody asks you the questions I am asking you, you should say that we didn't say what was going to be said?' (as cited in Brennan & Brennan 1990).

Misunderstandings can best be avoided by keeping sentences short. A short sentence is usually a simple sentence. Short, simple sentences tend to be easily understood because they avoid the following:

* Awkward phrases, especially complicated past-tense verbal

phrases (e.g. might have been), which are difficult for a young child to understand. To a preschool child, something either happened or it did not—the idea that something in the past might have happened seems silly. How to pose questions while avoiding such phrases is outlined in Chapter 3.

- Frequent use of pronouns (he, she and they) makes it difficult for a child to keep track of who or what is being discussed. It becomes a memory test for the child if the proper names of people, places and objects are not being used.

- Using too many embedded clauses (i.e. clauses within clauses, of which the lawyer's question cited above is a good example) can also put a strain on the child's memory. A child may find the sentence very difficult to follow and it will break up the flow of any conversation.

Question form

The form the question takes also influences the answer. Concrete questions, such as 'what', 'where' and 'who' questions, may be understood by the age of three. However, questions beginning with 'why' or 'how' can be difficult for any child to answer (Saywitz 1995). A child may not be able to consistently answer 'why', 'when' or 'how' questions until five or six years of age, as these questions tend to ask for more abstract, conceptual-type information. Further, 'why' and 'how' questions can appear very accusatory and may seem to imply blame. For example, 'How did that happen?' implies the child may have had something to do with, or had some control over, what happened. These questions, therefore, should be used cautiously with children of all ages.

Questions that require a 'yes/no' response only (see Chapter 3) are particularly problematic when adult concepts are being used. This is because the child's answer does not indicate to the interviewer whether he understands the question or not. A child may say 'yes' merely because he thinks that this is what the interviewer wants to hear.

Asking questions in a developmentally appropriate manner is one of the most challenging tasks for interviewers and it may therefore be helpful to do some further reading on this issue. There are numerous reviews that focus on the use of language when interviewing children, including Aldridge and Wood (1998) and Walker (1994).

Box 1.7   Try this

Below is a list of phrases that police officers and lawyers often use when they are interviewing children. Have a go at rephrasing each of the phrases so that a five-year-old child would be able to understand them more easily.

Tell me about that in more detail . . .
I'd just like to pause the camera while . . .
Are you aware that . . .
Can you describe the man . . .
Can you clarify whether . . .
You said earlier . . .
In reference to . . .
Your mother alleged that . . .
State your name . . .
Speak about the matter concerning David . . .
Subsequently . . .
I'd like to ascertain . . .
In regard to the bathroom incident . . .
At approximately . . .
I put it to you that it was later . . .
When did it commence . . .
Can you clarify . . .
Please indicate . . .
I know it is difficult to explain . . .
Suspect . . .
In sequence . . .
Please elaborate . . .
Talk me through the incident . . .
Observe how I . . .
What is your current address?
Report . . .
Take a written statement . . .
Matter . . .
Acknowledge . . .
Now I'd like to review . . .
Witnessed . . .
The occasion of . . .
Tell me the facts . . .
His age . . .

> Did you hear the conversation . . .
> Let me rephrase that . . .
> View this photograph . . .
> Prior to his arrival . . .
>
> You will find our suggestions in Appendix 1.

It is important to remember that a child is usually seeking to make sense of a conversation even if the question asked does not make sense. For example, in a study by Hughes and Grieve (1980), children between the ages of five and seven were asked a series of bizarre questions, such as 'Which is bigger, yellow or red?' Most children answered by attempting to apply some form of logic to the question—for example, yellow is bigger because that yellow cushion is bigger than the red one. One might reasonably wonder why children do not reply 'I don't know'. However, research suggests that even when a child is given the option to say that he does not know the answer, he may not choose it (Moston 1987). A child may assume that if an adult asks him a question it must be answerable. This was apparent to Stern (English translation 1939) at the turn of the century:

> To many witnesses a question acts as an imperative: 'You must answer'. They dare not confess their ignorance. Even when they start with an 'I don't know' they may be unable to maintain it against the insistence of an inquirer who repeats his question, hammering it home in persistent phrases.

As Hughes and Grieve (1980) concluded:

> Psychologists and linguists—and all others who rely on questioning young children—can no longer treat the child as merely a passive recipient of questions and instructions, but must instead start to view the child as someone who is actively trying to make sense of the situation he is in—however bizarre it may be.

2

PREPARATION AND PLANNING OF THE INTERVIEW

When interviewing a child, it is very important to have a clear indication of any special needs of that child before the interview begins. This allows you to adapt the interview accordingly. Sometimes finding the time to plan the interview properly may seem impossible. However, too often the worst interviews are those that were not planned.

WHY IS PLANNING SO IMPORTANT?

> *Box 2.1   Try this*
> Imagine you are about to interview a famous person you greatly admire. You are the only person who is allowed to speak with this person and it will be their last public interview. The interview will be televized around the world. Write down how you would prepare for the interview. What do you need to know?

If you had the choice of interviewing the famous person in Box 2.1 either straight away or after you had time to prepare for the interview, which option would you choose? Why? The same answer and reasons should apply when interviewing children. Preparation is important for thinking about all the issues that need to be discussed with the child, for preparing suitable questions and for being aware of fruitful leads to follow. While preparation takes up valuable time, practise makes more effective planners.

WHAT DO I NEED TO CONSIDER?

When planning the interview there are three main issues to consider that will help you decide the questions to be asked. These are: clearly understanding the main purpose of the interview; knowing as much as possible about the child's general background; and having some understanding of the personal details of the child.

Purpose

It is important when deciding on the purpose of the interview to fully understand what the present concerns or issues are and what gave rise to them. Obtaining more information surrounding the concerns is therefore useful. For example, you may wish to consult the child's parent or teacher about how the child initially talked about the event (if relevant), and how the parent or teacher interviewed the child about the event (they usually do). If the child has not spoken directly about an incident then you may want to know what behavior or events made the parent/teacher suspect abuse. However, keep in mind that any information you obtain from these sources may not be accurate.

When you were doing the task in Box 2.1, you probably knew exactly what you wanted to achieve from your interview (apart from international fame, of course). This helped you to decide what you would focus on and what you considered essential to know. For similar reasons it is useful to be clear about the purpose of an interview with a child. Understanding the purpose is essential for deciding which types of questions and interviewing techniques will be most effective.

Child's background

As you set about the task in Box 2.1 you probably wrote down what background information you needed to know in order to get the interest of that famous person in particular: who they are;

where they come from; what sort of language they use; what their temperament is like; what things they enjoy doing; what aspects of their background you're particularly interested in. All of these points are equally relevant for a child. For example, you may want to gather information on the child's age, developmental stage, linguistic ability and attention span. Again, information on these issues can be obtained from the child's parent or teacher. Such information is likely to have an important bearing on the interviewer's expectations for the interview. Table 2.1 (on p. 26) sets out a checklist of the aspects of a child's life you may find useful to learn about before an interview. It is a good idea to adapt this list to your own needs and to have it handy when preparing for interviews.

At first glance it might seem that obtaining all the information in Table 2.1 is unrealistic. However, if you talk to the parents or the child's teacher about how the allegation arose, you can use this opportunity to ask questions about other aspects of the child's life. Further, if you conduct a pre-interview assessment of the child (see later in this chapter), you can usually ask the child most of these questions before the interview. In particular, do not underestimate the usefulness of knowing the names of all the significant people in the child's life (including pets). It is very easy for the interviewer to misunderstand who the child is referring to—in one memorable case, the interviewer actually mistook the family dog and his licking habits for the child's father.

Personal details

It may also be relevant to know the child's likely words for sexual body parts, the family style with respect to privacy, nudity and bathing, and the expression of loving relationships in the family home. Further, it may be useful to find out about any possible contact the child may have had with sexually explicit videos, acts, TV shows or magazines, and whether the child has a sexually active older sibling in the home. These factors can explain why a child might display sexual knowledge beyond her years.

ARE THERE QUESTIONS I CAN PREPARE IN ADVANCE?

You do not know precisely what information a child has to tell, and so this will limit the number of questions that can be planned

Table 2.1 Information checklist for preparing an interview

1. Name of child:
      Nickname or preferred name:
2. Address:
3. Date of birth:
4. Legal status:
      with family: No/Yes   Names of people in household:
      in care: No/Yes   Type of care order:
5. Ethnic origin and religion:
6. Is there a problem with the child's ability to speak English?
      No/Yes, explain:
7. Does the child have any psychological or mental impairments?
      No/Yes, explain:
8. Does the child have any physical impairments?
      No/Yes, explain:
9. Type of suspected or known abuse (if applicable):
      Physical / Sexual / Neglect / Other:
      Description of injury:
      Medical examination required No/Yes, name of doctor:
10. Details of people important to the child:
      Name   Age   Amount of contact with child
        Mother:
        Father:
        Co-habitee:
        Other children:
        Aunt(s)/Uncle(s):
        Grandparent(s):
        Friend(s):
        Babysitter(s):
        Schoolteacher(s):
        Family pet(s):
11. Names of places where the child spends time:
      Address   Approximate amount of time spent there
        Home:
        School:
        After-school care:
        Babysitter's:
        Relative's:
        Friend's house:
        Other:
12. Significant activities that the child likes to engage in:
        Favorite school subjects:
        Favorite television programs:
        Favorite computer games:
        Favorite sports:
        Favorite books:
        Other favorite activities:

Table 2.2 Some relevant points to cover in an interview

1.	What is the likelihood that the behavior (e.g. abuse) actually occurred?
2.	Exactly what is the behavior?
3.	When does the behavior happen?
4.	How long does it go on for?
5.	How often does it occur?
6.	How severe is the behavior?
7.	Where does the behavior occur?
8.	What happens just before the behavior?
9.	What happens just after the behavior?
10.	Who is sees it happens?
11.	Who knows about it?
12.	How does the child understand the behavior?

in advance. However, if you know the main topic of discussion and the purpose of the interview, then it can be helpful to write down some possible lines of enquiry. For example, if a case of sexual abuse is suspected, the following areas might be considered:

• First, if it is a criminal offence that is being investigated, then it is a good idea to either create a list of questions relating to the legal points that need to be proved or to at least know what these points are.
• Second, if you know the type of abuse or the incident that occurred it may be helpful to have a list of questions prepared suitable for the age of the child and covering aspects you know will come up. For example, think how you might question a ten-year-old about bruises found on her body apart from 'How did you get those bruises?'
• Third, it may be useful to generate a list of possible explanations or hypotheses for the suspicions, disclosure or behavior that might need to be explored in the interview.
• Finally, in anticipation of establishing that the child *is* being abused, it may be helpful to jot down ideas about what information will need to be covered with the child to fully understand the nature of the abuse.

Table 2.2 offers a checklist of points that could be followed, whatever the subject of the interview is, to give you a guide for obtaining relevant information. These questions are not intended to be asked directly of the child, but rather to help you assess your progress in obtaining the information.

DO I NEED CONSENT FROM PARENTS TO INTERVIEW A CHILD?

For the sake of the child, it is extremely important to work with the child's supporting parent(s). If the parents are cooperative, it increases the likelihood that the child will be also. The best way to obtain the cooperation of the parent(s) is to keep them fully informed of your actions at all times and to ask for their permission before you interview the child. The procedures of the interview (and the need to ask highly specific questions) may also need to be explained to the parent, as well as the reasons why the interview is being recorded if this is the case. If the interview is to be videotaped, then the parent(s) could be shown the video set-up at the same time as this is shown to the child.

However, there are a number of situations where parental consent may not be sought or obtained. For example, a police officer may interview a child as a witness to a criminal offence without seeking parental consent. Legal consent is a complex issue so local legal and procedural guidelines should always be consulted (e.g. in the UK the guidelines include Home Office and Department of Health *Memorandum of Good Practice on Video Recorded Interviews with Child Witnesses for Criminal Proceedings*; Department of Health *Working Together Under the Children Act 1989. A Guide to Arrangements for Inter-Agency Cooperation for the Protection of Children from Abuse*; and Crown Prosecution Service *Code of Practice on Child Witnesses*).

It is also important to seek the child's consent (or assent) to being interviewed. Although the interview may be compulsory, obtaining the child's consent first will help build the child's trust. Further, if the child does not wish to be interviewed, it can be very helpful to know the reason why at the outset.

Box 2.2   Try this
Design a written consent form for parents and for an older child (i.e. over eight years of age) for an interview you wish to videotape. Think what information you need to include. Don't forget contact names and details in case the parents need to discuss matters further. You will find our suggestions in Appendix 1.

WHAT DO I TELL PARENTS WHEN THE POSSIBILITY OF ABUSE IS RAISED?

Many parents become highly anxious when first learning that their child might have been abused. At a time like this they may desperately seek reassurance and support from professionals who have had experience in the area. Care needs to be taken, however, not to fuel hysteria. A child can be very sensitive to anxiety in her parents and, in turn, become very anxious herself.

It is best to tell parents that, whether the child has been abused or not, they need to stay calm and be ready to support the child by listening to her when (and if) she wants to talk about the abuse. Trying to force their child to talk about it, while understandable, is not helpful for the well-being of the child. If the child does spontaneously talk, parent(s) should make a discreet note of what was said, and how, when and in what context it was said. The same goes for any unusual behaviors. Such information may be useful for determining the full extent of what happened to the child. Parents should also be reminded not to talk about the case in front of their child, or to reward the child for giving the interviewers information. Such behavior may encourage the child to inaccurately report events.

WHAT IS THE BEST INTERVIEW ENVIRONMENT?

The best interview environment is one that is uncluttered, comfortable, warm and friendly (possibly with a few bright children's posters on the wall to make the child feel at ease). If the child feels threatened or anxious, any reduction in formality may alleviate this. Try to have seating available that is appropriate for the size of the child. If possible, you should sit at the same level as the child, with your chair facing the child's chair at a slight angle. This is because if the child is seated beside you (e.g. together on a sofa), or is seated directly opposite you, she will not be able to (or want to) maintain eye contact for long. Instead, she will tend to sit and look at her feet, which may reduce the audibility of her account (Wilson & Davies 2000).

The interview room itself should be an airy, private environment that is free from unnecessary interruptions or distractions. Therefore, all technical equipment should be checked to establish that it is working before the child's arrival. The microphone (if it is to be used) is an exception as it needs to be checked using the child's voice so that the volume can be adjusted appropriately.

If the child appears to be overly anxious, distractible or uncomfortable, you will need to ask yourself—or the child—'What can I do to make this easier for you?' Flexibility is an important quality when interviewing any child.

Sometimes the interviewer will wear a uniform and this may intimidate the child. However, each child reacts differently to courtroom wigs and gowns or police officers' uniforms. One child may find the dress intimidating and recall less as a result (e.g. Powell, Wilson & Croft in press), while another may enjoy the authority the dress represents, feeling safe in the knowledge that she is being taken seriously. Sometimes the type of dress can turn the interviewer into a comical figure. For example, one eight-year-old child was very happy to be interviewed in court by a lawyer in a wig and a gown—she laughed and said she had never seen a man in a 'curly wig and black dress' before! It is important to remember that whatever the style of dress, competent interviewing is more likely to influence what a child says.

> **Box 2.3   Try this**
> Think back to the last job or course interview you attended. Think about what the interviewer(s) was wearing, the room layout, the questions that were asked, the timing of the interview and the general rapport you had with the interviewer(s). Did the interviewer(s) make you feel at ease? Why? Why not? What effect did this have on your performance in that interview? What could the interviewer(s) have done to improve your performance? Why is this important to you?

SHOULD I USE TOYS IN AN INTERVIEW?

The usefulness of toys, puzzles and stationery depends on how distracting they are and what they are being used for. Allowing a child to play with toys can be a good way to ease her into the strange interview environment. However, if the toys are too exciting, they may distract her. Getting a child to settle down and talk after an exciting game can be very difficult. For a nervous child, doing a quiet and relatively easy task together (e.g. a jigsaw puzzle or a card game) may help her to talk by deflecting the main focus of attention away from herself. However, make sure the activity is age-appropriate. The child may be offended if she is invited to play a game that she considers herself too old for.

Drawings can also be helpful, as most children like to draw. Having a young child draw a person and label the parts of the body can be a useful means of learning what names the child has for various body parts.

SHOULD I USE A SET OF ANATOMICALLY CORRECT DOLLS?

Dolls were first introduced into the interview setting to help children disclose abuse by decreasing reliance on their verbal abilities, and to aid memory. They were also introduced as a way of diagnosing abuse; it was assumed that abused children would play differently with their dolls from non-abused children (Kate, Schonfeld, Carter, Leventhal & Cicchetti 1995). However, research following the introduction of these tools has revealed that dolls do not always help a very young child to recall events they have experienced and they do not reliably discriminate the play behavior of abused and non-abused children (Goodman & Aman 1990). They can also be distracting. To use a doll or prop as a memory aid, a child needs to recognize that the doll can be a symbolic representation of herself (DeLoache & Marzolf 1995). The symbolic representation of objects, however, does not develop until at least six or seven years of age. Evidence for this can be seen in young children's play. A five-year-old girl who plays with a Barbie doll will rarely think that the doll represents her—she is more likely to pretend that she is Barbie. Until more research is conducted, it is better to avoid the use of anatomical dolls, particularly with a young child five years old or younger (Bruck, Ceci & Francoeur 2000).

WHEN SHOULD THE INTERVIEW BE CONDUCTED?

One of the most consistent findings in the research literature is that memory decays over time (Baddeley 1990). The longer the interview is delayed, the less likely that the child will remember details. If the child is being abused, then the longer the delay, the greater the possibility that the child will be exposed to further abuse and threat of harm. For these reasons, the interview should be conducted as soon as practical. That said, the interview should not be rushed or conducted if the child does not want to talk. One of the most frequent complaints from child interviewees is that they are rushed (Wade & Westcott 1997). Ultimately, the critical decider on whether an interview is conducted must be the child. No matter how urgent the case may appear, if the child is not willing to talk then an interview will be useless.

Careful consideration also needs to be given to the place and the time of day in which an interview is conducted. Conducting the interview during a child's nap time, mealtime or after the evening meal is rarely appropriate. Further, taking a child out of class can be very embarrassing or annoying, as the child's classmates may want to know the reason for the absence. Try to avoid scheduling the interview at times that may result in cancellation or a change in schedule. Where abuse is suspected, the interview should be conducted at a time when the suspected abuser will not find out about it and at a time when a trusted adult can attend. If facilities are needed that are only available on weekdays, this may be difficult.

> **Box 2.4 Try this**
> You have been asked to interview a seven-year old child who is in hospital. Where would you do the interview (she can move out of her bed)? Why? When do you think would be the best time? Why? What information do you need to answer these questions? How would you obtain that information? You will find our suggestions in Appendix 1.

WHAT SHOULD I DO WHEN I FIRST MEET THE CHILD?

First, you need to explain who you are, what your role is and why the interview is taking place. The same applies to other people in the interview team. Neutral descriptions of your job may be appropriate, for example, 'I listen to children who have worries . . .', 'I help kids sort things out . . .' The approach taken, however, will obviously depend on the child's level of understanding and on the circumstances of the concern.

Second, you should give the child a rough idea of what you will be doing together—that is, merely talking—and how long this will take. The child is likely to have little experience of interviews and may be concerned that she is in trouble (or will be for talking to you).

WHY DO AN INITIAL (PRE-INTERVIEW) ASSESSMENT?

A pre-interview assessment should be done by asking open-ended questions that allow the child to talk about innocuous events such as a school trip or birthday party. This gives you the best sense of the child's ability to recall past events and through this her style and the level of detail she can provide. It also indicates her level of development and temperament so that you can adequately plan the main interview and phrase questions appropriately. In addition, open-ended questioning helps you to build rapport with the child and to familiarize her with a style of interaction that is child-centered, that is, one that encourages the child to talk as much as possible. Subsequently, this may increase the amount of information that the child provides spontaneously (Sternberg et al. 1997). The potential benefits are so great that interview protocols, such as the Stepwise Interview (Yuille 1991) and the US National Institute of Child Health and Human Development protocol (Lamb, Sternberg & Esplin in press), recommend that the child is given practise in recalling two innocuous events that have been experienced before being formally interviewed.

Finally, a pre-interview assessment should also introduce the child to the ground rules of the interview (see next section) and give her an opportunity to demonstrate an understanding of these before relating any abuse-related information (Sternberg et al. 1997).

WHAT ARE THE GROUND RULES OF THE INTERVIEW?

A young child is often inexperienced in interviewing and does not appreciate the intent or purpose of an interviewer's questions (Siegal 1991). When a child does not understand the process or rules of the interview, she is less likely to provide a detailed account. Keeping the child informed of the ground rules of the interview lets her know the level of detail that is expected and how to behave in the interview. The child cannot learn such rules from anyone else. The ground rules used in the home and

33

classroom are likely to be very different from those of an interview. Taking the time to teach these ground rules is likely to pay off, because if the child understands the purpose of the questions there is a greater chance the answers will be relevant and useful.

Some of the most important ground rules for the investigatory interview are presented in Table 2.3. In the left-hand column is an example of what might be said to a child. In the right-hand column are explanations of the ground rule or a description of the rule in more detail. You may need to explain some of these (depending on the type of interview and the needs of the child) at any time during the interview process although, as mentioned earlier, it's best if you can go through them with the child before the interview.

Box 2.5   Try this
Write down the ground rules for a discussion about a science project between a teacher and a five-year-old child. If the child is asked a question by the teacher that he is unsure of, is he permitted to guess the answer or make it up? Does the teacher already know all about the science project? How does the teacher usually check and correct for any misunderstanding? Does the teacher need to know specific details about any information, like where or when the child learned it and who else was there when he learned it? Who is considered to have the expert knowledge about the project—the teacher or the child?

Compare your answers with the ground rules of interviewing that are laid out in Table 2.3. You will find our suggestions in Appendix 1.

DOES TELLING A CHILD TO SAY 'I DON'T KNOW' OR 'I DON'T UNDERSTAND' WORK?

In reality, when a young child does not understand a question, she is much more likely to try to answer it the best she can than tell the interviewer she doesn't understand. This is true even when she has a good rapport with the interviewer and has been encouraged to say 'I don't know' or 'I don't understand the question' (Moston 1987).

While Table 2.3 offers some useful suggestions for minimizing

Table 2.3 Some important ground rules of the interview

Ground rule	Elaboration
If I misunderstand something you say, please tell me. I want to understand everything you say.	It needs to be stressed to the child that the interviewer does not know what has happened and that if the interviewer says something that is wrong, the child has the right to correct him or her.
Please remember that I was not there when it happened. The more you can tell me about what happened, the better. So tell me everything you can remember, even things you don't think are important.	A child does not normally know what level of detail is required so it may be useful to explicitly state that anything he remembers could be useful. If you have time before the interview, allow the child to practice reporting as much as he can about an innocuous event first should help e.g. 'Tell me everything you can remember about having breakfast this morning, even things you don't think are important', 'Tell me more about what you ate', 'Tell me more about the kitchen'. Always explain clearly to the child why you are doing this.
If you don't understand something I say, please tell me and I will try to say it using different words.	Sometimes a child will tell an interviewer that he does not know the answer to a question when in fact he does not understand the question. Telling the child that you do not mind rephrasing questions may alleviate this problem somewhat.
It's okay to say 'I don't know' or 'I don't remember' to questions I ask.	It might be helpful to give the child some practise at doing this before the main interview, with examples of things they do know and things they do not know.
If you cannot remember everything, that's okay. Please don't guess. Just tell me what you do remember.	Often a child may be able to remember part of some requested detail but not all of it. The interviewer will want to hear what the child can remember, even if it is not the 'whole answer'.
Even if you think I already know something, please tell me anyway.	Often a child doesn't like to repeat information if he thinks an adult knows the information already.

Table 2.3   (cont.)

Ground rule	Elaboration
I promise I won't get angry or upset at you for anything you say.	The child should be explicitly informed that the interviewer will not be shocked or upset by what the child has to say because this may prevent the child from disclosing details (particularly on sexual matters).
It's okay to use any words that you want to.	A child may need to be told that he can use sexually explicit language. However, be prepared for it when he does. It can be shocking to hear such words as 'cunt' or 'prick' come out of the mouth of a young child.
It's important to only talk about things that really happened.	This is not a competency assessment (see Chapter 1 for a discussion on competency), but merely advises the child to speak the truth.

misunderstandings in the interview, the child may not respond to these even though she has understood them. The interviewer needs to be responsible for constantly checking the child understood the question and is answering appropriately (see Chapter 3 for questioning techniques). While the child should be informed that it's okay to say she doesn't know an answer, the onus is always on the interviewer to use simple language and to correct for any misunderstanding.

> *Box 2.6   Try this*
> Design a pre-interview assessment for the child in hospital (Box 2.4). What would you assess? What toys or props might you bring with you? How would you explain the process to the child? Which ground rules would you explain to the child during the assessment? You will find our suggestions in Appendix 1.

WHO IS THE BEST PERSON(S) TO INTERVIEW A CHILD?

Preferably only one person should be asking a child questions. A child can find getting to know even one interviewer stressful so the more interviewers she has to get to know the more stressful the situation can become. And the more stress a child experiences, the less detailed information she is likely to provide. For similar reasons, the same interviewer should conduct any further interviews. This provides a better opportunity for a trusting relationship to be developed with the child.

If possible, ask the child if she would prefer a male or female interviewer. Sometimes a child will feel more comfortable with either a male or female interviewer. In cases of abuse, a child may have strong preferences on this and it might help rapport if these preferences can be met. Sex is an important consideration when choosing an interpreter (see Chapter 4) as well as an interviewer.

SHOULD A SUPPORT PERSON BE PRESENT DURING THE INTERVIEW?

A child may want a support person to be with her during an interview. (In some jurisdictions, a support person is a requirement during a legal interview.) If a support person is present during the interview then it is important to advise him/her not to interrupt the child and not to ask questions or prompt answers. The obvious exception to this would be if the support person were also the interpreter. However, such practice is not advisable, as an interpreter needs to be impartial (see Chapter 4).

It is a good idea to seat the support person behind the child to limit the influence and possible distraction he/she may have. If the child appears uncomfortable talking about the abuse in the presence of the caregiver, or if the caregiver appears overly upset hearing about the abuse, then another person may need to be used who does not have a close interest (i.e. a neighbor or community worker). This may seem unfair on the child, however, a child sometimes finds it more embarrassing and stressful to speak about certain topics, for instance, sex and family relationships, in front of someone she knows.

WHAT ABOUT VIDEOTAPING THE INTERVIEW?

It is an excellent idea to videotape any interview with a child. This can allow you to have a permanent record of what the child said; to evaluate your interviewing technique later; and to have evidence should anyone dispute your conduct during the interview (unfortunately, this is more common than most people think).

In some areas it is now a requirement to videotape interviews with a child that form part of a sexual abuse investigation. This is so that the videotape can be shown in a court of law as the child's examination-in-chief and the interview, therefore, becomes evidence in a trial. (Often these tapes are used in civil and family courts as well.) If this requirement is the reason you are conducting a videotaped interview, you will need to consider local legal and policy guidelines regarding the creation and storage of a videotape. These tend to vary between countries and states. In addition, we recommend the following five minimum prerequisites to conducting such a videotaped interview:

- First, consider whether the child is capable of being cross-examined in a criminal court and would be considered competent to testify. If the answer is no to either or both of these questions, then submitting the videotaped interview to a criminal court may be unrealistic.
- Second, know how to use the video equipment effectively. If in doubt, have a technician check that the equipment is functioning normally. There is no point in conducting a videotaped interview if the child is not visible or her evidence cannot be heard. It may also be appropriate to check that your video equipment is compatible with the courtroom equipment.
- Third, ensure the picture and sound quality of the tape are adequate. Changes may need to be made to the interview room or the choice of where the interview is to be conducted to accommodate this. To minimize background noise, the room should be carpeted, situated in a quiet location (e.g. not near toilets or busy traffic areas) and contain low-noise furniture and furnishings (polystyrene chip-filled beanbags, for example, are not a good idea in this respect). To maximize picture quality make sure the room has curtains on any windows (closed curtains can produce a more even light). To ensure that the child is in the frame of the camera, the room needs to be relatively free from distractions so that the child is encouraged to sit still and talk rather than move around the room and play. The best camera angle is that which puts the child's face clearly into the frame.
- Fourth, carefully consider where the microphone should go. Often interviewers check their equipment using their own

(adult) voices. However, a child who is being interviewed about sensitive matters often sits with her head down and mumbles into her chest. It would be insensitive to correct a child for doing this when the child is disclosing a distressing event. The better alternative is to have a radio microphone that clips onto the child's chest. If the child mutters into her chest, the microphone can clearly pick up what is being said. If a clip-on or radio microphone is not available then be sure to test the microphone on the child's voice before the interview begins and gently encourage the child to speak up in response to initial questions.

- Fifth, if recording the time and date is not a standard feature of the equipment, it may be useful to purchase a generator that inserts this into the picture. If this is not possible, a clear-faced clock with a second hand visible to the camera can be just as useful. This demonstrates that the videotape has not been edited and can be very helpful if editing is required. Oral statements of the date and time can be made at the beginning and at the end of the interview to confirm that whichever device is used is accurate. This can be quite disconcerting for the child, though, so always explain to the child that you are going to do this in advance.

After the interview is completed, check the quality of the recording so that any inaudible words can be transcribed while the interview is fresh in your mind. When doing this, you can also make a quick index of the tape so that sections are easily accessible when you or others come back to review it at a later stage (for more comprehensive guidance on videotaping a child's evidence, see Wilson & Davies 1999).

Having said all that, there are some cases when video- or audiotaping a child is inappropriate. A child who has been involved in video or film pornography may find being videotaped very traumatic. If a child is distressed or uncomfortable with being videotaped then it is best not to use such equipment.

SHOULD I GET THE CHILD'S CONSENT?

Every effort should be made to obtain the child's consent to having the interview recorded (see Appendix 1, Box 2.2). In obtaining full consent, the purpose and procedure of using the recording equipment needs to be explained fully to the child. A young child may be concerned that her videotape will appear on television so she may need some reassurance about this. If the child asks whether the recording will mean she will not need to testify in court, explain that the court may require the child to give evidence anyway. However, unless the child raises the issue of court directly, it is best avoided. Most cases will not go to court. Further, the thought of testifying may create undue anxiety in the child, as can the hope of a prosecution that never eventuates.

HOW SHOULD VIDEOS BE FILED AND STORED?

Using one tape per interview makes the interviews more easily accessible. If limited space is a problem, try transferring the tapes to CD-ROM as they are more compact and last longer. Videotapes may not last for more than ten years unless they are re-spooled.

Since confidentiality is an important issue, it is advisable to store the tapes or CD-ROMs in a secure area so that they cannot be accessed by unauthorized personnel. The possibility of un-authorized access to the tapes should always be considered if tapes are copied. For example, there have been cases where tapes of children's interviews have ended up on the Internet. If possible, therefore, allow professionals to view the tape on site rather than taking a copy away with them. The fewer copies there are of a tape, the easier it is to keep track of them.

3

ESSENTIAL ELEMENTS OF THE INTERVIEW

The main exercise in any interview is to encourage a child to talk about certain topics. The best interviewers are those who listen a great deal more than they talk. The main interviewing skill is knowing how to encourage a child to talk honestly by asking questions that stimulate the conversation. This chapter presents a number of techniques that are designed to help you stimulate conversations with a child.

I AM A GOOD LISTENER BUT WHAT QUESTIONS DO I NEED TO ASK?

It is very easy for an interviewer to think that the main purpose of interviewing is to ask the 'right' questions. Indeed, an interviewer's main source of panic is that he or she will be unable to come up with *any* question let alone the right one. Questions are certainly important and poorly asked questions can definitely hinder an interview. However, often an interviewer can ask the child a stupid or inappropriate question merely to have him ignore the question and report exactly what the interviewer needed to know. This is because the child wanted to talk about what had been happening to him anyway. Using minimal prompts instead of questions can be the best way of showing a child that he is being heard, and this is what matters most to a child in an interview (Prior, Lynch & Glaser 1994).

> *Box 3.1   Try this*
> Sit still for five minutes and try to do nothing but listen. Close your eyes if that helps. Listen to all the noises around you. While you are doing this try not to think of anything else except the noises you hear. Try not to daydream or think about what you need to do once you stop listening. Also try not to analyze or converse with yourself about the noises, just listen to them. Try to do this for the full five minutes.

When you tried the exercise in Box 3.1 you may have had trouble concentrating. Often, trying to sit still and just listen is very difficult as the mind gets bored and drifts off or focuses on other things. Listening is a very powerful skill and one that can be learned (see Boggs & Eyberg 1990 for more detail on listening skills). Most people assume that they listen because the concept of having a conversation where no one listens would seem bizarre. However, in Western society, we quickly learn that the purpose of listening is primarily to know when it is our turn to talk again (which is usually about oneself!). A good interview, in contrast, is one where the focus of conversation is on the child.

> *Box 3.2   Try this*
> Spend one lunchbreak with a friend or colleague in which you practise listening. You are not allowed to talk about yourself or give an opinion or any advice. You are only allowed to ask about them and to listen to them. That is all. Be warned—this task is harder than it sounds.

WHAT DOES IT MEAN TO BE CHILD-FOCUSED?

Being child-focused means taking the child's perspective, allowing the child to do most of the talking and allowing the child's needs

Table 3.1 Suggestions for testing alternative explanations

---

1. If the child makes unusual claims, pursue them, don't ignore them. Ask the child to elaborate or explain what she means. There may be a logical explanation.
2. Gently check what the child means when she uses adult terms and concepts. At the end of the interview, review what the child has said while encouraging her to correct any misunderstandings in your summary.
3. If the child was not directly involved, ask the child if she actually saw what happened as opposed to just thinking or hearing that it happened.
4. If the child chooses not to repeat remarks stated previously, ask the child why she doesn't want to talk about it again.

(Adapted from Ceci & Bruck 1995.)

to be the main priority. This requires an acceptance that the child's needs may be different from your own. For example, suppose a child is being interviewed about possible abuse and he starts to say something but then stops abruptly. Many interviewers in this situation would feel the need to encourage (or pressure) the child because they believe that the child is concealing something and that encouraging him to talk would be in his best interests. However, this is not necessarily so. First, in many cases you don't know for certain that the child *is* being abused. Second, putting undue pressure on the child may result in a disclosure but it may not be the right one. That is, when a child is put under pressure he may say anything to get out of the situation (as adults often do). Third, even if a clear and accurate disclosure is obtained, this forced disclosure may not leave the child feeling better. For example, some interviewers pressure children by claiming that the alleged offender will be sent to jail, hence the child will be safe. However, very few disclosures result in a jail sentence for the offender. Further, there is little evidence that arresting or locking the offender in jail (particularly if the offender is a parent) is in the best interests of the child. Sometimes it certainly is and, as anyone who has worked in child protection knows, sometimes it is not. The point is that it is important to respect a child's wishes even if they sometimes clash with the interviewer's. After all, the child is the one who has to cope with the consequences of any or no disclosure.

WHAT DOES IT MEAN TO BE OPEN-MINDED?

To be open-minded means that the interviewer is open to any possibility regarding what happened to a child. Regardless of what background information you have, there are numerous possible explanations for the concern. Abuse is only one of them. Even when there are medical findings or other evidence to suggest that the child has been abused, it is important not to jump to conclusions until all information has been collected and, where possible, validated. While in such cases it is *likely* that the child was abused, there have been situations where a far less sinister explanation for the concern was revealed. Different possible explanations should therefore be gently explored, without pressuring a child to provide the information that you require. Table 3.1 provides some suggestions for exploring alternative explanations of a circumstance with the child. It is always a good idea to map out two or three different explanations yourself beforehand that you may wish to explore in the interview.

Another characteristic of open-minded interviewers is that they do not judge a child or burden him with their personal feelings of anger, disgust or horror. Instead, a general air of acceptance of what a child is saying should always be maintained. This is important because a child can be quick to pick up any inflection in the voice of approval or disapproval of the answer just given. Interviewers who are open-minded show they support the *child* rather than what the child *is saying*.

WHICH INTERVIEW PROTOCOL SHOULD I USE?

There are numerous very good child interview protocols available (see Poole & Lamb 1998 for a review). If you are a child-protection professional, your departmental agency (or local legislation) may offer clear guidelines on which protocol to use. Most of the popular interview protocols (e.g. the *Memorandum of Good Practice*, the Stepwise Interview and the Cognitive Interview) have the same essential stages and elements (see Table 3.2). Hence, if you are not constrained by local guidelines, it doesn't make much difference which protocol you use—they are all similar. In fact, they are so similar that it is very difficult to identify precisely which protocol an interviewer is using.

The structure outlined in Table 3.2 has several important features. It is child-focused because it allows the child to direct the interview as much as possible, and it maximizes the child's free narrative—that is, the child's report is obtained using prompts rather than specific questioning. Further, the structure places a

Table 3.2 Elements common to all standard interview protocols

Stage	Description	Clarification
1	Greeting and establishing rapport with the child	Pre-interview assessment is conducted and the ground rules are established.
2	Introducing the topic of concern	Purpose of the interview is explained and the key ground rules are re-introduced (or introduced if the interviewer has not already introduced them).
3	Eliciting a free narrative account from child	Child tells everything she can remember about the event. Interviewer uses general prompts and minimal encouragement to get child to report as much as possible before asking more specific questions.
4	Specific questioning	Specific questions are asked to fill in gaps, clarify details, or clear up apparent inconsistencies in child's account. Questions are kept short and simple and, in particular, double negative or complex grammatical constructions are avoided.
5	Closure	Interviewer summarizes child's account to allow child to correct any misunderstandings. Child (and any support persons) are debriefed and thanked for cooperation.

high priority on the establishment of a good rapport with the child (Stage 1). Finally, by opening with free narrative or general questions before moving to specific questions, the structure provides little opportunity for the interviewer to contaminate or manipulate the child's report.

Generally, the interview structure can be seen as a funnel where the interview begins with the most open-ended questions and progresses down to the more specific questions. In practice, it is easier to use this funnel approach for each topic, rather than for the interview as a whole. The structure is a guide only, with no set of specific questions you must use. One child will want to focus on the reason he is there and get his story heard. Another may be more reluctant and require more direct questioning (although always return to open-ended questions as soon as possible to reduce the risk of contaminating the child's report).

Let us then look at each of these suggested interview steps in turn.

HOW DO I START THE INTERVIEW?

You will probably have introduced yourself when you first greeted the child and he may know you from a pre-interview, but when you settle down to the interview proper, it is a good idea to state your name and role again. If you are audio- or videotaping the interview, then the date and time might also be mentioned here. This can seem odd to a child so either explain to him in advance that you are going to do this or avoid the situation altogether by using a timing device attached to the equipment. You also need to point out the recording equipment (if you have not already done so) and explain what it is there for—for example, 'We are recording this so that you do not have to repeat things for me' (see Chapter 2 for advice on recording interviews).

As a start to the interview you should reiterate the ground rules. Hopefully these will have been demonstrated or discussed at the pre-interview stage (see Chapter 2 for information on both the ground rules and the pre-interview). If not, take the time to go slowly through them or the ones you consider most important at this stage. Throughout the interview the child may need to be reminded of some of these rules (especially during questioning). However, any competency-type questions should not be used again. Asking a child about truth and lies after he has talked about an incident can seriously undermine his confidence and emotional stability as it may appear that the interviewer no longer believes him (Wilson & Davies 1999).

> *Box 3.3   Try this*
> Write a concise paragraph (no more than fifteen lines) that introduces your name, the video camera (and why it is there) and contains the following ground rules:
>
> • To tell me everything you remember, even little things that you don't think are important.

- That it's okay to say 'I don't understand'.
- That it's okay to say 'I don't know'.
- Not to guess an answer.
- To remember I will not get angry or upset with you.

Write the paragraph as if you were speaking to a six-year-old child. Use Table 2.2 to help you. You may find it useful to memorize the paragraph so that you can use it in your interviews. This may help you to relax, feeling confident in the knowledge that you have mentioned everything and have started the interview smoothly as well. You will find our suggestions in Appendix 1.

WHAT IS RAPPORT?

In the interviewing literature 'rapport' can mean two different things. First, it can refer to the positive relationship that is crucial to develop between the interviewer and the child if the child is to trust the interviewer. Thus, 'a good rapport' means a strong element of trust between the child and the interviewer. The interviewer engages the child, is calm and helps him to feel relaxed and that he is listened to. As strange as it may sound, appearing to be overly sympathetic or concerned about the child can destroy rapport. A child can find anxious interviewers, and those passionately trying to support him, very intimidating. A child often experiences difficulty dealing with his own emotions during an interview, and it can be overwhelming trying to cope with the interviewer's reactions as well (Sattler 1997).

Building rapport involves listening to the child (Boggs & Eyberg 1990). In order to listen, you cannot be doing all the talking. To do less talking you must ask open-ended questions—'Tell me about your favorite television program?' Open-ended questions encourage the child to do the talking, thus building rapport. Further, any amount of time spent building rapport is likely to pay off later in terms of the amount of detail the child will subsequently provide. This is because the more comfortable the child is within the interview setting, the more information he is likely to share, particularly information that is perceived to be traumatic or embarrassing.

47

The second use of 'rapport' in some interviewing protocols is in the 'rapport phase' of an interview. Here 'rapport' refers to the period at the beginning of the interview where rapport-building is specifically done. This usually involves a five-minute discussion (using open-ended questions) about the child's favorite television programs, school activities or hobbies. Ironically, rapport can be destroyed during this phase if it is adhered to consistently. For example, in one case, when a child wanted to talk about the man who raped her, the interviewer kept interrupting her, telling her that they would get to that later. The interviewer then redirected the child to talk about her favorite television program and school activities, making the child become very upset. In this case the interviewer was more concerned about being seen to have conducted a 'rapport phase' than actually building rapport with the child. Building rapport requires listening to what the child wants. In short, if the child wants to chat, then chat. If the child wants to talk, then listen.

Building rapport should not be confused with being best friends with a child. In the same way, building trust should not be confused with creating a situation where the child becomes eager to please you. Research suggests that 'very warm and friendly' interviewers can increase the amount of both accurate and inaccurate details a child reports about an event (Ceci & Bruck 1993). This is because a child can be eager to comply with what he thinks a warm and friendly interviewer wants to hear. To avoid this, the interviewer should be accepting of any type of response the child provides (silence and 'don't know' responses included), and should avoid interrupting the child when he is talking. Again, open-ended questions are best as they encourage the child to talk without implying specifically what the interviewer wants to know.

A child with a short attention span or other behavioral problems may require praise and encouragement for engaging in the process of the interview. In such cases it is best to focus any praise on the child's behavior, that is, sitting still, thinking hard, rather than on the quality or content of the child's answers (see Chapter 4 on how to engage such a child in the interview process). When rapport is particularly difficult to establish, it may be useful to contact an adult that the child trusts. Ask the adult if he or she will recommend you to the child. This may help the child understand that he can trust you.

HOW DO I START THE CHILD TALKING ABOUT THE ALLEGED EVENT?

One of the best ways to start a child talking is to ask the child directly: 'Do you know what you have come here to talk about?' More than likely, the child will immediately disclose an incident without the need for more specific lead-in questioning other than the prompt, 'Tell me more about that'. If the child says 'I don't know' in response to this opening question, then try mentioning the event that gave rise to the interview. How you do this will depend on the type of incident that is suspected. Table 3.3 provides options based on where the initial information came from.

Note that in the first option the interviewer is not asking the child to repeat what the child '*told* mummy about Uncle Joe', but rather 'what *happened* with Uncle Joe'. This is an important distinction. You do not want to know what he told the parent, only what actually happened. Also note that in the third option, a young child is unlikely to have any idea 'how' he got a disease. In this case, you may need to go back a step and ask him about his normal routines (and any variations or unusual events in his routines) to find out what has been happening to him.

WHAT IS FREE NARRATIVE?

A free narrative account is 'free' in that the interviewer has not helped the child construct it. The interviewer has allowed the child to talk as much as possible before specific questions have been asked. Free narrative is considered to be the most reliable component of an interview, provided the child has not previously undergone highly leading or suggestive questioning (Ceci & Bruck 1993). During free narrative, the child might be confused about the temporal sequence or may merge information from separate occurrences of the behavior; however, he is less likely to make something up or guess to please the interviewer. This is because open questions used to obtain free narrative do not specify the type of information that is required, and they do not offer information that may be incorporated into the child's later accounts. For this reason, the child's free narrative stage is considered crucial. Lucy McGough, a US researcher, cleverly relates this to the Humpty Dumpty nursery rhyme: once you've lost the

Table 3.3 Explaining the purpose of an interview to the child

Initial suspicion	Example of interviewer's question
Something child has said	'Your mummy said you told her that Uncle Joe upset you. Did you tell your mummy Uncle Joe upset you?' If child says 'Yes', say, 'Tell me what Uncle Joe did that upset you.'
Adult's suspicion about a place or person	'Sandra told me that you get upset when Uncle Joe comes to stay at your house. Is this true?' If 'Yes', 'Tell me what made you get upset.'
Physical signs or disease	'Do you know how you got that sore there?'
Change in the child's behavior that may indicate symptoms such as anxiety, depression etc.	'Your mummy told me you've been very scared at night. Have you been scared at night?' If 'Yes', 'Tell me what you've been scared of.'

opportunity of obtaining a free narrative before specific questioning, she suggests, all the best judges and lawyers in the world can never put the child's account back together again (McGough 1994).

HOW DO I ENCOURAGE A CHILD TO GIVE A FREE NARRATIVE ACCOUNT?

At first, it can appear to be very difficult to encourage a child to talk freely about something he either does not want to discuss or something he thought he had given enough detail about (e.g. 'He just messed with my bum'). An evaluation of police interviewers in the United Kingdom reported that in 43 per cent of interviews, the child was needlessly rushed from free narrative to the questioning phase (Davies et al. 1995). There are numerous possible reasons for this. First, the level of detail that is required when conducting a police investigation can pressure police officers to focus and seek clarification too soon on every comment the child makes. Second, conducting an interview with a young child that may later be used as evidence in court can be an anxiety-provoking task and anxiety tends to make interviewers rush through the process. Third, a child tends not to provide much detail in his free narrative. While an older child will provide more than a younger child, it can appear that free narrative probes do not elicit much information relative to what can be obtained using multiple specific questions.

The good news is that the art of obtaining a detailed free narrative from a child is something that can be learned with practise. It requires patience, the ability to tolerate silences and to hold one's tongue when the desire for a specific detail arises. Non-verbal prompts (such as 'mmm', 'really', 'oh', and gentle head nodding) can be used to mildly steer the child to the next point in the report. General open-ended questions, such as 'Tell me more about that' and 'What happened next?', can also help. Further, repeating two or three words of what the child has said can stimulate further conversation from the child. For example, a teacher conducted the following interview to find out how an eleven-year-old child assaulted a nine-year-old child in the playground.

> Teacher: Tell me exactly what happened.
> Child: He just came over, right and he just bashed this guy's head in. The guy's a psycho.
> Teacher: He just came over . . .?
> Child: Yeah, I mean he was like, going on and on, saying stuff, like, you know, 'I'll show you, you dick', then he was swinging his arms round and kicking him and everything.
> Teacher: Swinging his arms around . . .?
> Child: Yeah, like this [child demonstrates], he was like, standing on top of the poor guy and yelling.
> Teacher: [nodding] Ah-ha.
> Child: I mean John tried to pull him off and give him back his knife. I wouldn't of, I would have kept it. He's such a psycho . . .

This example shows the power of free narrative. If the teacher had taken the child's first sentence as his whole statement, and then asked more specific questions, the child might have been reluctant to mention what the fight was about. Initially the child implies that there was no reason for the attack ('He just came over', 'He was like, going on and on'). However, as the interviewer encourages the child to keep talking, it becomes apparent that the assaulted child may have stolen a knife from the other child.

For a teenager who knows exactly why he is being interviewed and wants to talk, these techniques are usually successful in extracting a great deal of information. The teenager will understand what type of information to give and will know what to say. A younger child, on the other hand, is more likely to expect the adult to structure his report for him and to correct him as he speaks. He is also less likely to understand what information is required and how to put this information into a coherent sequence. Therefore, it is important when you are interviewing a young child to be patient and to let him talk at his own pace without interruption. Specific questioning should not begin until you are certain that the child has completed his account or will not volunteer any more information.

HOW DO I KEEP A YOUNG CHILD TALKING?

A young child does not tend to say much at any one time, and it can take a lot of skill to keep him talking. In fact, the younger the child, the less likely a detailed account will be obtained spontaneously (see Pipe & Wilson 1994). However, it is younger children who are the most vulnerable to the contaminating effects of leading and direct questioning (Ceci & Bruck 1995) and who therefore need the most encouragement to provide a free account.

Here are a few tips that may be useful:

- When you ask the child for more information, try to avoid questions he can say no to (e.g. 'Did anything else happen?'). A child tends to see this type of question as a prompt to stop the interview, similar to asking, 'How are you?', to which you are supposed to say 'Fine', end of conversation. It is better to imply that there is more information: 'And what else?' or 'Tell me more about that'.
- Try to avoid asking any specific questions while the child is providing his free narrative. You do not want to break the flow of the narrative, and any interruptions to the child's train of thought will probably limit the amount of information he provides. Make a brief note of any specific questions so that you will remember to ask them at a later, more appropriate time in the interview.
- Do not underestimate the value of non-verbal prompts. If you sit and nod as you are listening to the child then stop nodding, the child will see that as a cue to stop as well. If you keep comfortable eye contact with the child, the child will keep talking. If you gaze out the window, the child may stop talking. Adults normally mirror the body postures of those they are talking to if they like them. Sometimes it may be appropriate to mirror the child's body posture or part of it. For example, if the child is drooping the shoulders, you may try doing the same.

- Let the child have physical space. This is very important if you are large, as you can appear to 'overcrowd' a young child in a small interviewing room. Make movements slowly—nod slowly, move in your seat slowly (if you need to) or relax slowly back into your chair. If you relax and take your time, the child will be encouraged to do so as well.
- If the child gives only a short account (e.g. 'We went to the party, we ate and then we went home'), encourage him to keep talking by going back to a part in the narrative and ask for further details ('A party? Tell me more about the party'). These prompts are important because they are general. That is, while they focus the child on a particular part of his account, they do not dictate what specific information is required.
- If the child is a preschooler with limited language, see Hewitt 1999 for other methods to encourage and communicate with the child.

Box 3.4   Try this
Spend an hour with a child. Ask him about anything (a trip to the beach, what he did yesterday). Try to keep him talking without asking specific questions. Use phrases like 'tell me more' and non-verbal prompts like nodding. And enjoy it. It's hard work but it can also be very amusing, especially the look on the child's face when he realizes you just want to keep him talking!

WHAT ARE OPEN-ENDED QUESTIONS AND WHEN DO I USE THEM?

Open-ended questions are questions that do not make assumptions or assume a particular answer, and encourage more than a two- or three-word response. The questions usually take the form of requests for more details about events already mentioned by the child; hence they usually follow, or are part of, the initial free narrative stage of the interview. Examples of these questions include, 'Tell me more about the time you were in the park' or 'I didn't understand that bit about the tickling game. What were you doing again?' or 'Before you said you don't like bath time.

53

Tell me more about that.' The phrase 'Tell me' can sound demanding, so it is important to ask it in a tone that suggests you are merely interested to hear more. Many interviewers try to soften the phrase by asking, 'Can you tell me . . .?' However, this is not advisable because the child is highly likely to respond to a 'Can you . . .?' question with either a yes or no answer. In contrast, 'Tell me . . .' assumes there is more to tell. It is important, of course, to remind the child that it is okay to say 'I don't remember' or 'I don't know' because there may actually be nothing more for the child to tell.

When phrasing questions, it is essential to use the child's terms, even if the child has used obscure terms for parts of the body or for any object, event or person. If the child's language is corrected or questioned, then he will feel he is 'getting things wrong' and there is increased risk of confusion and misunderstanding. If you do not understand a term the child has used it is better at this stage to let the child continue and to save your request for clarification later. This may seem odd—if you don't understand someone you normally tell the other person straight away. However, doing this can interrupt the flow of what the child is saying and often you can guess what the child means by the context. For example, 'He was tickling me on my icky, I told him to stop and he said he would, he gave me a packet of potato crisps, he did'. The best question to ask next is, 'Tell me more about the tickling' rather than stopping the child and asking, 'What do you mean by "your icky"?' While it is important to establish the child's meaning of this word, this can be done later.

Box 3.5   *Think about this*
Imagine you are the interviewer in the following situation:

Interviewer: What happened when you went into his bedroom?
Child: He hurt me, he hurt me bad, I told him to stop but he didn't.

What is your next question? Here are two alternatives:

Version 1:
Interviewer: Who hurt you?
Child: John.

Interviewer: Who is John?
Child: Mum's boyfriend.
Interviewer: Okay, how did John hurt you?
Child: He pushed down and got on top of me.
Interviewer: What did he push down on?
Child: The bed.

Version 2:
Interviewer: Tell me what happened.
Child: He pushed down and got on top of me.
Interviewer: He got on top of you . . .?
Child: He put his hand up my rudey and . . .
Interviewer: And . . .?
[Pause]
Interviewer: It's okay, take your time
Child: He took out his willy, he did . . . and he hurt me lots.

Which version do you think builds the best rapport? Which one allows the child to talk freely? Version 2 is the better alternative as it allows the child to keep talking. Although the details required in Table 3.4 might not be disclosed without specific questions, it is generally true that the more you allow the child to talk, the more details the child will report spontaneously. The more details the child reports spontaneously, the fewer questions you will need to ask later.

WHAT SPECIFIC DETAILS DO I NEED TO COVER WHEN DISCUSSING PHYSICAL/SEXUAL ABUSE?

If you are not qualified to interview a child specifically about sexual abuse, then listen to what the child has to say, thank the child for talking to you and contact your local child-protection agency. If you are qualified to interview the child about such matters, once the child begins talking about the abuse, try to obtain the information set out in Table 3.4 by using simple, non-leading questions. However, be aware that the child may not be able to remember or describe many of these highly specific features. Even adults find it hard to report events in this manner.

Table 3.4   Details required for report of abuse

1. Information about the exact nature of the incident or alleged abuse. For example, 'Tell me what happened', 'Let's talk about that some more. What exactly was Joe doing in your bedroom?'
2. The alleged offender's identity. For example, 'What did Joe look like?', 'Where does Joe live?' or 'What was Joe wearing?'
3. The length and frequency of abuse. For example, 'How many times have you done [the behavior] with Joe?', 'Did you do it one time or more than one time?', 'When was the first time it happened?'
4. The location and approximate date and time of the abuse (see Table 3.6 for further points). For example, 'When did [the behavior] happen?', 'Was it a school day or a home day?' or 'Do you remember anything special that happened around that time?'
5. The existence and location of any physical evidence, e.g. photos, clothing, video equipment, bedding and lubricants. Try: 'Tell me what you saw in the room.'
6. Anything the offender might have said to the child during the abuse, including threats, coercion or rewards. For example, 'What else did Joe say to you?'.
7. The location of other people. For example, 'Who was in the room when it happened?' or 'Was there anyone else in the house?'.
8. Who the child first told, where she told it, and what she said. For example, 'Who did you tell about Joe touching you in the bathroom?'.
9. Whether the child knows of any other victims and potential witnesses. For example, 'Were there other people in the bathroom?' or 'Has Joe touched other children?'.

When asking for specific details about abuse, try not to focus too much on the painful parts of the child's account, particularly if the child appears to be distressed talking about these. If the child appears to be upset, give him a moment or two to relax. Alternatively, allow him to take a short break to gain composure (if this is requested). This would also give you the chance to sit and think for a few minutes while you get your questions clear and concise in your mind before starting the interview again. While it may be difficult for the child to talk about the abuse, in encouraging him to do so try not to appear as though you are overly eager for him to talk about it. Avoid cheers like 'Great job' or 'It is good to tell'. The best way you can support the child is to listen and show him that you have heard what he said.

Alternatively, rather than take a break, if things get too distressing, you could change the topic to less traumatic aspects of the event—'I can see you're getting upset. Would you like to talk about something else for a moment or two? We can come back to this later.' This allows the child to relax a little before moving back onto the painful parts of his account again. However, if you do this, always clearly explain why you have changed the topic. The child may think you want to change the topic because talking about the abuse is not acceptable. Also, the child may not want to change the topic, but would rather get it over with.

If you are a child-protection professional, consider making two recorded interviews when a child reports that there are other victims. The first recording would explore the abuse committed against the child and the second what the child knows about abuse involving other victims. The second recording is essential for the investigation but, due to its hearsay nature, may or may not be admissible in court. Clearly explain the reason for the second interview to the child. For example, when he starts to talk about other children, allow him to finish his statement and then say you would like to hear more about that later on, as you need to know clearly what happened to him first.

WHAT ARE SPECIFIC OR DIRECT QUESTIONS AND HOW DO I USE THEM?

Specific questions are questions that ask for precise information. As such, they usually require only a few words in response. For example, 'Who shot the gun?' or 'What time of the day was it?' These questions focus the child's attention on a narrow or specific aspect of the event that may need to be clarified but would not otherwise be provided during the child's account of the event. There are numerous points for which precise information may be needed. You may need to obtain information regarding the nature and context of the event, for example, 'Where were you when Joe touched your bum?', 'Where exactly in the bathroom were you?', 'When you were on the toilet, what was Joe doing to help you?' Specific questions may be needed to clear up inconsistencies or misunderstandings in the child's account—'What were you wearing? . . . Pyjamas . . . What was Joe doing with the nightie, then? . . . Whose nightie was it? . . . Where was Sarah when this was happening?' Specific questions are also needed to clarify terms the child has used—'What did you mean when you said you "went down on" Joe? . . . I'm not sure I understand what you mean by "a golden rainbow".'

While specific questions can be useful (Davies, Westcott & Horan 2000), you should use them cautiously. Error rates increase with the use of these questions compared to open questions and general probes (Ceci & Bruck 1995). Specific questions can offer cues that help prompt the child's memory. However, if the details requested are not clear in the child's mind, he is likely to confuse the event with other events, or make something up just to please you (Hughes & Grieve 1980). Minimizing the number of specific questions, therefore, will minimize error in the child's account. Remember, however, the potential for error is not entirely related to the specificity or type of questions that are used. The type of language you use and the complexity of grammar will have a large impact on the child's ability to answer a question.

WHAT ARE CLOSED QUESTIONS AND WHEN DO I USE THEM?

Closed questions are a form of specific question because they focus the child on the specific information that is required. With closed questions a child has a very limited range of answers, usually two. While these questions put less weight on the child's verbal ability, they are most likely to lead to errors as they simply require a yes/no response or the child to choose between various choices provided by the interviewer. For example, 'Did this happen in spring, summer, autumn or winter?', 'Was your mum with you when you watched the TV?' For this reason, most protocols discourage the use of closed questions (Peterson & Biggs 1997). Nevertheless, there are strategies you can use to minimize error. Following each closed question with an open-ended prompt (e.g. 'Tell me more about that') allows you to check that the child has understood your question and is not merely saying something to please you. Also, if you limit most of your closed questions until the end of the interview (after as much spontaneous material has been gathered as possible), you reduce the risk of contamination.

WHAT ARE LEADING QUESTIONS AND CAN I EVER USE THEM?

Leading questions are those questions that suggest a certain answer is desired or assume the existence of facts that have not yet been proved or have not already been mentioned by the child. For example, 'Daddy hurt you, didn't he?' when the child has not yet claimed Daddy did anything. Suggestive questions include any questions where the interviewer's tone, manner or phrasing indicate that a particular answer is desired. For example, 'Are you talking about Paul, John . . . or is it JOE?' Common leading and suggestive questions in interviews specify the alleged offence or offender before the child has stated it. For example, 'Tell me what Joe did to you' when the child has not yet indicated that Joe was the offender, or 'Did Joe touch your front bottom or back bottom?' when the child has not stated that Joe touched him in either area.

A common misunderstanding among interviewers is that questions are suggestive only in their content rather than their context. This is not true. For example, if five of the first ten questions in an interview are about the alleged offender, this would be considered suggestive. This is because such questioning creates a situation where the child knows what the interviewer wants to hear about, even if the interviewer didn't directly state that this person had done anything wrong. Indeed, an interviewer can be suggestive without asking any questions at all. If eye contact and praise increase when a child talks about the alleged offender, this would signal that this is an area the interviewer wants to hear about, and the child would naturally focus on that particular area of content. Further, just repeating a question can be considered very intimidating and leading. For example, 'Just tell me where Uncle Joe touched you . . . Go on, tell me . . . Where did he touch you? . . . It's okay, just tell me.' This would be considered coercive even if the child *had* already mentioned that he was touched somewhere by Joe.

Of all the questions put by an interviewer, leading and suggestive questions are the most likely to result in errors in the child's account (particularly in young children, that is, those below six years of age). For this reason, leading questions should be avoided where possible (see Ceci & Bruck 1993 for discussion). However, it may *not* be possible or even advisable to avoid them completely. A leading question may be used for information that is not related to the abuse (for example, confirmation of the child's name and address). Further, if a child who is suspected of having been sexually abused will not acknowledge (in response to non-leading open questions) that anything occurred, it may be useful to state the source of your suspicions and ask the child whether the information is true. For example, 'Your mum thinks someone may have hurt you. Has anyone hurt you?' If the child says 'Yes', then the interviewer can immediately return to open-ended questions such as 'Tell me about that.' Note that normally it would be inappropriate to use the term 'that', as it is vague, but here it is unknown what the specifics are, and it is not appropriate to follow a leading question with another one.

It is a common fear among interviewers that if they do not ask leading questions, they will not be giving an abused child sufficient opportunity to talk. While this may be true in some circumstances, leading questions do not necessarily give frightened or embarrassed children the opportunity they want. After all, the crime committed may not be the one that you are suggesting. Further, leading and suggestive questions can be intimidating for a child. Taking the time to create a good rapport with the child is likely to be more fruitful for you and more comfortable for the child than resorting to leading and suggestive questions.

That said, leading questions about abuse allegations are sometimes asked among a series of questions, most of which do not relate to abuse. Take, for example, the case of a ten-year-old boy who has been physically abused, with numerous deep cigarette-burn marks on his arms. He appears to be developmentally delayed and is presently sitting in his hospital bed with the covers pulled up to his face. He is sucking the corner of the sheet. He does not appear to want to talk. The interviewer decides to ask a series of questions along the following lines:

> What do you call this part of the body? (Interviewer points to head.)
> Has anyone ever hurt you on the top of your head?
> Tell what happened when your head was hurt.
> What is this part of the body called? (Interviewer points to eyes.)
> Has anyone ever hurt your eyes?
> Tell what happened when your eyes were hurt.
> What is this part of the body called? (Interviewer points to nose.)
> Has anyone ever hurt your nose?
> Tell what happened when your nose was hurt.
> What is this part of the body called? (Interviewer points to mouth.)
> Has anyone ever hurt your mouth?
> Tell what happened when your mouth was hurt . . .

(See Appendix 1, Box 1.4 for the full transcript.) The interview proceeds in the same format as above with shoulders, arms, hands, chest, tummy, back bottom, front bottom, legs and feet, in that order. This approach could also be used with a picture of a person or a gingerbread man.

There are a number of positive points to note about this style of interviewing. First, because the interview has a clear rhythm to it, the child usually enjoys taking part. Second, the child can easily pick up what is coming next, as there is a consistent format to the questioning. Third, no aspect of the child's life is being focused on exclusively, hence the child knows the interviewer will quickly move on to another area. This style of interviewing is a form of the protocol called SAGE, Systematic Approach to Gathering Evidence (see Roberts & Glasgow 1993 for more detail). Its technique may be suitable for those children who will not talk (due to developmental or emotional reasons), or who require direct questioning because of their mode of communication (e.g. augmentative and alternative communication users, see Chapter 4).

HOW CAN I PHRASE QUESTIONS TO MINIMIZE ERROR IN A CHILD'S ACCOUNT?

Table 3.5 summarizes some of the best recommendations for using questions effectively.

CAN I REPEAT MY QUESTION?

There are two situations when an interviewer may want to repeat a question: when the interviewer needs to clarify what the child has said; and when the child did not appear to understand the question the first time. In neither situation is it helpful to repeat a question word for word.

At those times when you need to clarify what a child has said, clearly explain this to the child. For example, in an interview with a ten-year-old sea scout, the interviewer misunderstood what the child was saying. He asked for clarification in the following way:

> Child: The boat was out at sea but . . . the boat is actually more of a yacht.
> Interviewer: I'm not sure I understand, you said the boat was out at sea but you said the boat was actually moored at a dock?

If the interviewer hadn't realized at the time that he had misunderstood the child, he could have come back to it later by saying, 'I want to ask you about the boat again because I did not understand you the last time. Where was the boat when Joe started touching you?'

Some interviewers can unintentionally make the interview seem like a test of what the child knows (with the focus being on the child's performance) rather than taking responsibility for obtaining and understanding information. Always let the child know why

Table 3.5 Using questions effectively

1. Emphasize to the child that it's better to say 'Don't know' than to give an answer that she is not sure of.
2. Be careful not to ask questions that a child is not capable of answering. For example, do not persist with highly specific questions about details such as clothing, appearance or details about a room.
3. 'Why', 'when' and 'how' questions should be avoided with children below six years of age. This is because they require abstract concepts and reasoning skills that children don't acquire until they are much older (see Chapter 1).
4. Mix specific questions with open or general probes to avoid the interview sounding like a test, and follow up a closed question with 'Tell me more about that' or 'How do you know?' to check that the child has not made up a response to please the interviewer. For example:
   Interviewer: Did Joe hurt you when you were in the house?
   Child: Yes, in the bedroom.
   Interviewer: Tell me as much as you can remember about what happened in the bedroom.
5. Speak slowly and clearly, using short, simple sentences that contain no more than one question. Try to avoid the use of passives and negative questions. Ask 'Did you see Joe', not 'Was Joe seen?'; and 'Did you tell anyone about this?' not 'You didn't tell anyone about this, did you?'.
6. Watch carefully for signs of confusion and blankness and assume responsibility for clarifying the child's understanding of the questions and for cleaning up inconsistencies in the child's account.
7. Use the child's own language where possible.

you are asking the question again. Rather than asking, 'Can you explain that again?', try saying, 'I don't quite understand, I'm a bit slow today', or try to repeat the child's own words with an air of interest—'He hurt you?' This is more natural and it indicates that you genuinely want to understand what the child has said and want to know more, rather than you don't accept or believe the child.

If it appears that the child does not understand the question, repeating it word for word will not help. Try to rephrase the question, simplifying the grammar or the concepts used. For example, in this interview a medic was asking a seven-year-old child about his injuries. The boy had fallen off his bike (damaging the bike) and his parent had violently assaulted him for his 'stupidity'. The medic was trying to establish which injuries, if any, were caused by the parent.

> Medic: You mentioned that Mum got very upset about your bike getting damaged and that she hit you. Did you get those sores on your torso then or did they happen when you fell off your bike?

Child: Yes.

Medic: Why don't I try and explain that again! How did you get these sores [points to child's abrasions] on your tummy?

It is likely that the child had little idea what a torso was. All professionals have jargon that is peculiar to their profession and it is easy to accidentally use such terms when talking to a child. However, the grammatical construction was also a little too complex for a child, but the medic realized this and clarified the situation well. Notice she did not ask, 'Did Mum do this to you?', as that would be too leading. Sometimes it can be difficult to rephrase a question on the spot so you may need to come back to the topic later.

Be careful about repeating a question. A child often assumes that a repeated question is asked because he gave the wrong answer the last time and this may encourage him to change his answer to please you (Siegal 1991).

HOW DO I HELP A CHILD DISTINGUISH ONE EPISODE FROM MANY?

If you are a police officer, you should check your local legislation regarding what information needs to be obtained about repeat offences. In some areas, the child may need to remember the specific dates of various offences; however, in others, he may merely need to specify how long the abuse was going on for.

Remembering a specific occasion on which a repeated offence is committed is a difficult task, even for adults. While a young child (as young as three years) can report what usually happened in the event, he probably cannot provide many accurate details about one specific occasion. This is because memory tends to confuse or merge the many repeated events together (Powell & Thomson 1996). The younger the child, the greater the confusion, because a young child's knowledge of time and sequence and his ability to monitor sources of information are not well developed (Powell & Thomson 1997a). However, the appearance of errors in a child's report should not be taken to mean that the entire account has been fabricated. Table 3.6 offers a list of suggestions for helping a child to minimize errors and maximize the accuracy of specific details about an instance of a repeated offence. For more detail on this issue see Powell and McMeeken (1998).

Box 3.6 Try this
Katherine and her boyfriend, Tom, often look after Sarah (aged twelve years) and Mikey (aged six). They often babysit the children on Saturday nights. However, they are now suspected of doing more than just babysitting. Tom has previously been charged on eight counts of sexual assault of a child. However, he has never received a conviction for these charges. You are interviewing each child. How would you talk to them about the Saturday night babysitting sessions? How would you phrase the questions differently for Mikey? What information is relevant? You will find our suggestions in Appendix 1.

HOW LONG SHOULD I INTERVIEW A CHILD WITHOUT A BREAK?

The child should guide you on the length of an interview, as each child differs in his ability to concentrate and stay focused. Trying to push a child of any age who is restless and unable to concentrate will not help the interview content or your rapport with him. Normally, an hour is too long and much too long for a child who is a preschooler, developmentally delayed, hyperactive, anxious or distressed. However, if the child is given breaks when he needs them and he is willing, the interview may go on longer.

The timing of a break should be considered carefully. You do not want to disrupt a child's flow of thought, and a scheduled break that falls as soon as the child starts talking about an event may give the impression that you do not want to hear about it or that the child shouldn't have told you. It is a good idea to always ask the child if he would like a break rather than informing him that there will be a break in the interview. The child may prefer to keep going and to get the interview over with. If a child requests a break, it should be given immediately. The break should never be based on completing any part of the interview (e.g. 'We can have a break after you tell me about . . .') as this could be seen as bribery or coercion, especially if the break is needed to get a drink or go to the toilet.

That said, sometimes it is the interviewer who needs a break

Table 3.6   Maximizing a child's ability to discriminate between events

1. Record a child's statement as soon as possible after it is established that an offence may have occurred, and minimize the amount of questioning prior to this statement.
2. If a child has to give evidence after a long delay, she should be allowed to review her earlier recorded statements or partake in further interviews before the trial to refresh her memory.
3. Minimize the number of highly specific questions about a single instance of the abuse throughout an interview (particularly with children five years of age and below). Ask yourself whether you really need to ask a specific time-related question, or whether you can ask the question another way.
4. Conduct an assessment of a child's ability to locate events in time during the pre-interview phase. This can be done by checking with her caregiver the time and place of a significant event that was independent of, but occurred around the same time as, the alleged incident(s) of abuse (e.g. a birthday party or school outing). The interviewer can then question the child about this non-abusive experience during the rapport-building stage of the interview to determine the amount and quality of detail that the child can provide and her knowledge of time-related concepts. In the course of this, interviewers might be surprised to learn that the child does not fully understand common terms such as 'yesterday', 'tomorrow' and days of the week, even though she has been using these words spontaneously in her account.
5. Allow the child to report 'what usually happens' (with few prompts) before obtaining details about one or more instances of the offence.
6. When recalling separate instances of abuse, the child should be allowed to fully report one part of the incident or one full incident before moving on to the next.
7. Generate a unique label (using the child's own words) that allows each separate incident to be identified and discriminated from the rest. Examples of labels include 'The time in the bedroom', 'The time that Shannon slept over', 'the first time', 'The time when you watched the movie'. Contextual labels such as these are more effective than purely temporal labels (e.g. the second last time). When you have determined a label, it is important to consistently use that label when referring to the instance, otherwise confusion may result.
8. Offer the child frequent reminders about which incident is being reported. If the child provides new information, check that she is still referring to the incident or event that was just being discussed. For example, 'Before you told me that he gave you a funny elephant toy. Were you still talking about the weekend with Uncle Joe?' Such ambiguities can be clarified after the free narrative is exhausted.
9. Pinpoint the approximate time of each incident by helping the child to remember what was going on around the time of these incidents. For example, 'Was it a school day or a home day?', 'Whose class at school were you in when it happened?', 'Were you still living at your old house or had you moved by then?' It is easier for the child to remember the

context of an event than it is to work out whether the event occurred 'before' or 'after' another event (e.g. Christmas).
10. Focus the interview on the most memorable events or aspects. The first and last instances and any unusual instances (i.e. those that happened in a different place or manner) are likely to be the easiest to remember.

(Adapted from Powell & McMeeken 1998.)

to think through the next set of questions and how to ask them. Also, the interviewer may want to seek feedback or advice from colleagues. This is useful provided the breaks are timed carefully (i.e. during a natural break in the conversation), and the child is told the reason for the pause. If the interview is being recorded, then the reasons for any interruption should be carefully noted on the tape, together with a record of what occurred during any interval(s).

WHAT IF THE CHILD BECOMES A SUSPECT FOR A CRIMINAL OFFENCE?

Sometimes when a child is talking about sexual abuse, he may mention that he victimized another child or he may report some other criminal offence (e.g. stealing for the alleged offender). If the child is above the legal age of criminal responsibility (usually between the ages of eight to fourteen years, depending on the jurisdiction), he may be charged with an offence. This is a 'grey' area and the needs of the child must be of prime concern. It is a good idea to formulate a strategy with your colleagues for dealing with such cases so that everyone knows how they should deal with them. How you deal with each case will depend on how you balance the needs of the child, your role and the purpose of the interview.

HOW DO I END THE INTERVIEW?

Many interviewers overlook the need to properly close an interview. However, the closure is just as important as any other part of the interview. In particular, it has a large impact on the child's perception of the experience and his willingness to disclose information in further interviews. For this reason, a proper closure is important irrespective of whether the child disclosed anything at all.

First, the closure should summarize what (if anything) the child has talked about. This allows the interviewer to check with the child that everything has been understood by encouraging him to correct for any misunderstanding. If the interview was videotaped and the child's account is frequently clarified throughout, this may not be so important. Next, the interviewer should thank the child and allow him to ask any questions or discuss concerns he may have (see Chapter 5 on how to discuss potential concerns). It is important to explain honestly and in an age-appropriate manner what is likely to happen next and that there are a variety of consequences that may follow from an interview.

Third and finally, the interviewer should provide contact details for the child and the caregiver or parent to encourage them to make further contact if desired. Again, it is important for the child to know that he can come back to see you if he has more to say.

HOW DO I KNOW IF I NEED TO CONDUCT FURTHER INTERVIEWS WITH A CHILD?

The decision to conduct further interviews will depend on how much information the child has provided and whether the child is likely to disclose any further useful information in subsequent interviews. Rarely does a child exhaust all the information he knows in a single interview. Further, new information may come to light and the child may need to be interviewed again in order to clarify matters. For example, in paedophile cases, the alleged offender may have abused a number of children. One child may come forward and discuss what happened to him and his friend. The friend may mention another two children. One of the two other children may mention something happening to the first child that the first child had not mentioned.

It is important when conducting a further interview to provide the child with a clear explanation as to why he is being interviewed again. Otherwise, it might be interpreted as the interviewer not believing the child or the initial answers being wrong. Multiple interviews should not be conducted where the original concerns were vague and/or the child is clearly resistant to the interviewing process. Such situations can result in high levels of coercion and suggestive interviewing. Further, children report becoming very distressed at being interviewed multiple times as this can feel like an ongoing interrogation (Prior, Lynch & Glaser 1994).

4

TAILORING THE INTERVIEW TO THE CHILD'S NEEDS

The interviewing techniques outlined in Chapter 3 provide the standard basic procedure of any interview you conduct with a child. However, the application of these techniques is likely to be more demanding when the child has expressive or receptive difficulties, attention problems, feels self-conscious or is ill at ease in the interview. When this is the case, the child is more vulnerable to suggestion and the task of remembering is going to be a more challenging one for her. Thus, you will need to take more care when interviewing to ensure that she has the best possible opportunity to communicate what she can remember.

Although we all live in the same world, we all experience it differently. What contributes to those experiences includes our family history, our abilities and the culture we grow up in. Often we categorize our experiences as attributable to this religion or that cultural group or as a result of a particular age or a certain disability. The problem with categorization is that few people turn out to be typical of any given category, and this goes for children too. Take, for example, one child interviewee who had a Japanese mother, a French father and was brought up in the United Kingdom! The child didn't know what 'English' was—she spoke all three languages interchangeably not realizing they were separate languages (her mother did this also). This child may have been exceptional but each child has unique aspects that are important to consider when interviewing. Whatever the child's background, your main task is to listen and accept her, and this means doing all you can to understand her. (For further information than this chapter covers on disability and multicultural issues, see Braithwaite & Thompson 2000.)

WHAT ASPECTS OF A CHILD'S LIFE DO I NEED TO CONSIDER WHEN INTERVIEWING HER?

Your ability to communicate with a child will largely depend on your awareness of her family, cultural, intellectual or personal background. Knowing this will help you to establish rapport with the child, to ask developmentally appropriate questions and to understand the context and meaning of her answers. Table 4.1 outlines some of the main factors to consider when tailoring an interview to suit a child. Each of these factors is discussed in more detail in the remainder of the chapter. However, it should be noted that little research has focused on the effect of these factors when interviewing a child, so the recommendations we make are largely based on experience. Further, not all of these factors will influence each child in the same way. There are marked individual differences in the way people react to any given situation or background.

The best way to explore these factors is to speak to people who know the child well, such as a teacher or caregiver. However, you may still need to observe the child directly and listen to her responses in the interview context before deciding how best to tailor the interview to suit her needs. Again, flexibility and the ability to be open-minded, that is, to think about a variety of explanations for the child's responses or behaviors, are important qualities of interviewers.

If your initial interactions with a child suggest that there are numerous potential barriers to communication, it may be fruitful to spend more time getting to know her before you conduct the main interview. This is where the pre-interview can be particularly important as it will allow you to explore more effective ways of interacting. There is no value in conducting an interview if you cannot understand what the child is saying, or are causing offence or creating anxiety due to ignorance of cultural issues.

Table 4.1 Factors to consider about a child interviewee

Factor	Importance
Race, culture and ethnicity	Establishing rapport, in knowing how to communicate in a style that is meaningful to the child, and knowing how to interpret verbal and non-verbal responses; the child may prefer an interviewer of the same/different cultural group.
Sex of child	Determining whether a particular sex in interviewer is preferred.
Educational history and intellectual performance	Checking the child's communication abilities and limitations, including mental impairments.
Health and physical status	Checking the child's physical impairments; determining the effect any medication (or lack of) may have on the interview process.
Family background and parental relations	Determining the child's attitudes to people of your profession and degree of support from various caregivers; determining the family's reactions to the alleged offence, and the influence of these reactions on the child's willingness to disclose.
Siblings	Establishing the influence of older siblings on the child's knowledge and language.
Psychological status, personality and temperament	Establishing the child's level of stress in the interview, coping skills, and style of responding to questions.

HOW SHOULD I INTERVIEW A CHILD WHO CAN SPEAK ADEQUATE ENGLISH BUT IS FROM A DIFFERENT CULTURAL GROUP?

Assessing English proficiency is a difficult task because a child who appears to use English fluently in the rapport-building stage can have considerable communication difficulties later in the interview when the questions become more specific and detailed. The task of deciding whether an interviewer requires interpretive assistance is a difficult one (see next section on choosing an interpreter). Even if the child is truly bilingual, you may want to consider seeking the assistance of an interpreter. A bilingual child often uses a mixture of words or phrases from both languages and may not always know the precise English word to use. There may be other benefits to using an interpreter. For example, if the

71

child spoke a different language with the alleged offender, it would probably be easier for her to recall the abuse in that language. Further, translation is not merely about translating words, it also involves an understanding of the cultural significance and meaning of those words.

Regardless of whether you work with an interpreter or not, you should understand something of the cultural background of the child. Overall, there are four separate tasks in assessing this: identifying the cultural group the child belongs to; considering which aspects of the culture may be relevant to the child; assessing the degree to which the child and family identifies with this culture; and assessing how these factors may impact on the interview. (See Appendix 2 for references regarding different cultural groups.) Let us look at each of these tasks.

Identifying cultural group

The first task is to identify to which cultural group the child belongs. This should be done with some care. In some multicultural settings, there are a variety of groups which are easily stereotyped as being the same, even though they are not. For example, it is inappropriate to consider all people of Asian origin as 'Asians'. Although there are similarities in Asian cultures, there are important differences between them. This issue should also be viewed in light of possible tensions between groups based on current or historical issues (see Ponterotto et al. 1995 for a review).

Relevant cultural aspects

The second task is to consider which elements of the child's cultural background may be relevant. For example, are his religious beliefs or gender roles significantly different from your own? What historical/cultural factors may be important? What are the family's attitudes about the prevalence and effect of child abuse? How is authority viewed in that culture? Who is allowed to ask questions? What kind? How do people in that culture relate to each other? Are direct questions used to obtain information, as is the case in Western culture? Is eye contact expected when listening? Is touching or holding another a norm? Are there people within the community that the child is not supposed to talk with? How does a child within that culture view her elders?

Local agencies are likely to be of particular assistance in answering these questions and there are also books that address these issues. For example, Sattler (1998) offers a detailed description of the questions to consider in working with some minority groups. It is easy to stereotype and value certain aspects of a culture. So be cautious of this in the interview setting. It is also critical that you do not demonstrate a cultural bias by valuing your own culture more than the child's. If prejudice is likely to influence your behavior (regardless of whether it is based on real experiences), you should try to arrange for somebody else to conduct the interview.

Family identification

The third task is to assess the degree to which the child and family identifies with the culture. Often, a child may take on board more of the mainstream culture than that of her parents. A child is often more adept at moving between cultures than her parents and may place less emphasis on traditional cultural values and behaviors than her parents. This lower level of emphasis on traditional values can create tension within certain families, and such tension may influence the course of an interview, particularly if community elders are present. It is important, therefore, to assess which cultural values are relevant to this child's life and this situation.

Influence on interview

Finally, you need to assess what the important cultural elements in the interview situation are, and how these elements affect the interview process. For example, should the interviewer be someone from the child's cultural group? Is the way you are dressed likely to cause offence or anxiety? How does the child respond to people in authority? Is direct eye contact likely to influence the outcome of the interview? Has there been a history of dominance of your cultural group over the interviewee's that will lead to a particular style of response to your questions? Do the dolls or toys that you use have the appropriate cultural identity?

Box 4.1   Try this
Think about the predominant cultural groups in your area and try to answer the following questions about each of these cultures. How do they relate to each other? How do

they view police, social workers and other mental health workers? What is their attitude towards child physical and sexual abuse? Do the views of the family conflict with those of the state? What are some of the ways in which a failure to recognize cultural differences might lead to misunderstandings and misjudgments in the interview? Taking the above information into consideration, how would you alter the way you conduct an interview with a child of one of these cultural groups? Consider creating a list of agencies or people who could keep you informed on such issues for a diverse range of cultural groups.

WHAT NEEDS TO BE CONSIDERED WHEN CHOOSING AN INTERPRETER?

When choosing an interpreter, some general principles need to be applied and allowances may need to be made for different cultures.

First, it is recommended that a qualified or professional interpreter be used. Since you may not understand the comments made between the interviewee and the interpreter, it is important that you use an interpreter who is professionally trained and who fully understands the needs and demands of an interview. The interpreter must be aware of the importance of neutrality, strict translation (i.e. conveying equivalent tone of voice, body language and even using swear words) and must be prepared to come under your guidance at all times. An inexperienced translator may be shocked by what a child says and may not believe the child. The ability to remain impartial and to hide personal opinions about the child or the situation is a skill that is just as important for an interpreter as it is for an interviewer. For these reasons, while it may be tempting to use a relative or friend of the child as an interpreter (particularly if the language is not common), this practice should be avoided wherever possible.

Second, the gender and status of the interpreter may be an important issue to consider. For example, it is inappropriate in some cultural groups for a male interpreter to interview a female child about sexual assault, and vice versa (Powell in press). Further, a child may be fearful of speaking in front of a person of authority within the community. Indeed, there might be a genuine risk of the child being punished for her behavior or disclosures. It would be wise, therefore, to discuss these issues with the child as well as any possible interpreter before the particular interpreter is chosen for the interview. To offer adequate advice on this, however, the child and the interpreter will need to know the type of questions that will be asked. They may not anticipate that explicit and specific questions may be asked, particularly about acts of a sexual nature.

WHAT NEEDS TO BE CONSIDERED WHEN WORKING WITH AN INTERPRETER?

Interpreters can be used in many different ways, depending on the needs and the linguistic capabilities of the child. In some cases, most of the interview questions may need to be relayed through an interpreter, whereas in others, the interview could be conducted in English, and the interpreter only used to explain difficult concepts, such as the purpose or possible consequences of the interview.

The appropriate use of an interpreter requires the recognition that *you* are interviewing the child, not the interpreter. However, the interpreter has the responsibility to inform you when misunderstandings or potential communication problems arise.

The interview should be conducted in a way that does not isolate the child at any time. The seating should be arranged so that the interpreter is at your side, and so that you can maintain good eye contact with the child (if this is culturally appropriate). Further, you should always address the child in the first person when you ask a question. In other words, rather than ask the interpreter about the child, phrase your question as if the child can understand you. Even when asking for clarification about a response, you should always address the child, not the interpreter.

To minimize interpreter bias or misinterpretation, sentences should be kept relatively short and simple in structure. The interpreter's memory is not likely to be able to hold detailed information while performing the complex task of accurate translation. If you summarize what you have learned at various stages throughout the interview, it offers the child and the interpreter the opportunity to confirm and correct for any misunderstanding that may have arisen along the way.

If you have not used an interpreter before, it is a good idea to arrange to meet with the interpreter before the interview. This allows you to outline the interviewing procedure and to discuss the types of questions that will be asked. After you have completed the interview, meet with the interpreter again to discuss problems that were encountered in the process. An effective working relationship with an interpreter takes time to develop and if you ever get the opportunity to call on that interpreter again, you will both have a better idea of how to make the process easier. (See Sattler 1998 for a good discussion on working with an interpreter.)

HOW DO I ENCOURAGE A FRIGHTENED CHILD TO TALK?

It may not be helpful in situations where a child refuses to go into the room with you to use 'persuasion'. Attempts to convince the child verbally that there is nothing to worry about may increase the child's anxiety by focusing her attention on her fears and the strange interview environment. Further, if you are slightly anxious about whether the child will go with you, the child may sense this and perceive it as confirmation that there is something to fear. An alternative approach might be to immediately engage the child's attention (or rather, divert it from the strange interview environment). This can be done by showing her some interesting toys, objects or equipment, or by engaging the child in an interesting age-appropriate task or conversation. A confident, calm, friendly approach that assumes cooperation is likely to be most fruitful here. For example, this is how one interviewer successfully distracted a frightened four-year-old child when she first approached him in the waiting room:

> Interviewer: Hello James. I'm Cathy . . . I'm a police lady. I'm going to be talking to you for a little while this morning. [Interviewer immediately directs child's attention to a stuffed toy he is holding.] Wow . . . who is this you have with you?
> Child: [crying] My bear.
> Interviewer: Your bear! . . . and he's a very cute bear too . . . what's his name?
> Child: Boo [still crying].
> Interviewer: What a great name. Where did you get him?
> Child: I . . . I don't know . . . . Mum got him for me.
> Interviewer: Well, would Mum, Boo and you like to come and sit down . . . Perhaps you can tell me what you and Boo like to do together . . .

Note that the interviewer did not attempt to lead the child away from his mother. The child was already distressed, and this was likely to have made it worse. Once the child had entered the room and had calmed down, the interviewer then asked the mother to wait outside. However, before doing so, issues of safety and the expectations of the child were briefly addressed. The door was left slightly open and Mum left her car keys and handbag on the table to reassure the child that she would not be leaving without him. The interviewer clearly told the child that they were going to talk for half an hour while his mother waited in the waiting room. This introduction was effective because it made clear to the child that the interviewer was merely there to *talk* with him and it indicated where the parent would be during the meeting (Sattler 1998).

To help a child feel safe and to reinforce for appropriate behavior, it is important to provide clear expectations of what the child is to do in the interview (Sanders & Dadds 1993). A young child has little experience with formal face-to-face interviewing and may have misconceptions about what is expected. She may believe that you will take her away from her home or do something to hurt her. Also, a child who has low self-esteem or is frightened may be quite restless, demanding and distractible in the interview. Having effective strategies for engaging the child in the interview process, therefore, plays an important role in making her feel settled and secure.

The best way to help a young child to take part in an interview is to encourage appropriate behaviors, such as sitting still, listening to the questions, thinking hard about the answers, waiting patiently and speaking clearly into the microphone. Praise is useful as long as it is based on the child's behavior and *not* the content of the child's answers. In other words, you should provide reassuring and friendly responses to *any* type of answer (demographic, irrelevant and don't know responses included), not merely responses that are helpful and relevant to the purpose of the interview. Also, praise should be used early in the interview. It may be gently phased out as the child becomes more comfortable. For example, if the child says 'I don't know' in response to a question, encourage the child by saying, 'That's fine if you don't know'. Congratulate the young child for speaking clearly (for a tape recorder) by saying, 'That's a big voice, well done!' Praise the child who sits still, even if it is only for a few seconds, by saying, 'Thank you so much for sitting still, you must be thinking hard'. By encouraging the child's behavior, you are letting her know what is appropriate without scolding her. Other forms of disciplining a child during an interview (e.g. reprimanding her or raising your voice) may appear to work, but they are likely to destroy rapport.

Box 4.2 Try this

Write an introduction for a bright four-year-old child who is emotionally disturbed. Think about what you would say in words and your non-verbal behaviors. How would you encourage him to talk? Write your answers down.

Now answer the following questions: Is your introduction age-appropriate? Is age-appropriateness important in this case? Did you state your name and explain your role? Did you explain the purpose and structure of the interview, including your expectations of the child? Are your non-verbal behaviors helpful? What are the signs you look for in the child that indicate he has engaged with you and is ready to get on with the task of the interview?

You will find our suggestions in Appendix 1.

WHAT SHOULD I DO WHEN A CHILD BECOMES DISTRESSED DURING THE INTERVIEW?

A child can become visibly distressed or agitated during an interview for many reasons. Perhaps the child feels emotional pain associated with remembering the trauma or she is anxious about being in the strange interview environment. Perhaps the child is fearful of the consequences of disclosure, is tired of answering questions or is hungry. There are numerous ways a child experiences stress in the interview situation, and attempts to minimize this should be based on your best judgment about the needs of each child, taking into consideration the child's non-verbal behaviors and her developmental level. It may be useful to ask the child if there is anything you can do to help. She may want a short break, a glass of water or a tissue. She may want to continue and get it over with. Every child is different.

In cases where the child has experienced severe trauma, the child may demonstrate seemingly bizarre behavior as she appears to relive the event. This is called 'dissociation'. In such cases, the child needs therapeutic help and the interview should be discontinued. For example, during an interview in which a sixteen-year-old girl was discussing a series of sexual assaults carried out by her father, she began to scream at her father to get off her as she struggled to get out from underneath him. Her father was not in the room and no one was holding her down. Such cases are relatively rare, but it is always a good idea to have the name and phone number of a trusted therapist on hand to refer the child to if needed.

If the child breaks down and cries, it is important to remain calm and show that you are listening and accepting of her feelings. Further, you need to show that you have the patience and respect to allow her to express her experiences in her own time. If necessary, shift the questioning to a less threatening topic for a while, or have a short break while the child gains composure. Acknowledging the difficulty the child has in talking (e.g. by gently saying 'It's okay to cry' or 'It's hard to talk about these things') is a good way to demonstrate your empathy. However, empathy should not be confused with sympathy or overt demonstrations of concern. Empathy is letting the child know that you accept her feelings. Sympathy (and concern), in contrast, is telling the child *how* you feel about what has happened to her. As we have noted, it is never appropriate for the child to have to deal with your feelings (Sattler 1998).

Further, the interview is not therapeutic in nature. Attempts to ease the child's worries by reassuring her that it was not her fault, or that she has done the right thing by telling, may in some circumstances be detrimental to the child's recovery (see Chapter 5 for a more extensive discussion of this issue).

WHAT DO I DO WHEN A CHILD REFUSES TO BE INTERVIEWED?

There isn't much you can do. If the child refuses to talk, ask her if there is anything you could do that would make the process easier for her. If she still does not wish to talk, thank her for listening to you and for coming to see you. Always let the child know that you are happy to talk to her at a later date, if she wants to. A child who has been abused may need time to get used to the idea of being interviewed, as often initial disclosures are unintentional. Wade and Westcott (1997) asked children what prompted them to talk about the abuse and showed that disclosure to authorities was often accidental. Sometimes a child told her friends and her friends told others. Sometimes the abuse was discovered only after a child indirectly made reference to it. In these circumstances the children were not prepared to make full disclosures despite pressure from an interviewer. Such children may well come back at a later date to talk to you, so it is important to leave the door open for them to do so. Be careful not to judge a child merely because she does not want to talk about it straight away.

HOW DO I TAILOR AN INTERVIEW TO A CHILD WHO HAS AN INTELLECTUAL DISABILITY?

An intellectually disabled child is defined as a child who is over the age of five years and has significant subaverage intellectual functioning (as measured on IQ tests), as well as significant deficits in adaptive behavior compared with other children of the same age and culture (American Psychiatric Association 1994). In other words, a child with an intellectual disability may have problems with self-care, daily living skills, communication, social skills, personal independence, and may be more likely than her peers to exhibit difficulties with the use and understanding of speech and language.

Before the interview, you will need to check out with the child's carers what the particular skills and strengths of the child are. Further, ask them about the best ways to encourage and praise the child, as well as the child's likes and dislikes—rapport is crucial if you are to keep the child's attention.

There is large variability in the cognitive, communicative and social development skills of intellectually disabled children, so it is important not to underestimate the child's abilities in the early stages of the interview. You should always begin interviewing the child as you would a child or adolescent without an intellectual disability; that is, use clear, simple language, words or concepts that the child is familiar with, and use broad open-ended questions where possible.

During the initial stage of the interview, you need to determine the child's preferred method of communication and start thinking about ways you can accommodate this. Does the child communicate with verbal speech only or does she use a combination of speech and gesture? Does she use an augmentative system such as an electronic aid or a communication board/book that contains symbols and/or photographs? Allow the child plenty of time to respond to your probing, using whatever method she finds most comfortable. Be careful not to talk over or provide words for a child who has difficulty speaking. The key is to be patient and let the child speak for herself. You can help her do this by remaining responsive to her communication abilities and limitations and being flexible enough to alter your questions and strategies when needed in the interview. She may, for example, rely on extra visual cues to understand what has been said. She may also have other physical impairments, including hearing problems and vision problems, and she may be easily distracted (refer to sections on these aspects below).

If you have not understood what the child has said to you, tell her that and ask her to say it again. As we have said before, if you repeat the question without telling the child that you have not understood her, she may assume that the first answer was not appropriate or correct. If you still experience difficulties, you could ask the child to slow down or to 'show you' with the assistance of mime (natural gesture), an object, augmentative system (if she has one) or pictures. Alternatively, the child could be encouraged to write a word or draw a concept, to try using alternative words, or to spell the word. If you still do not understand what has been said you may have to resort to closed or yes/no questions to narrow down and eliminate the possibilities of what the topic is. However, these questions should be used with caution as a child with communication or intellectual disabilities may be particularly susceptible to interviewer suggestibility and may say yes to yes/no questions just to please you (Milne & Bull 1996). If this appears to be the case then it may be better to use an interpreter to help you interview the child (see previous section in this chapter on how to use an interpreter—the same principles apply). Unfortunately, in this type of situation there might be no alternative but to use the parent, carer, guardian or someone who knows the child well as interpreter because few others may understand the child's idiosyncratic use of language. The obvious danger in using an acquaintance as interpreter with severely disabled children is that one of the few people who understand and have access to the child may be the one who is abusing her. It is useful to find out from more than one carer of the child how the child might communicate aspects of the abuse. By doing some research in advance, you may require less assistance in understanding the child than you originally anticipated.

Echolalia is a term used when the interviewee answers with what you have said word for word. An example of this is when a child is asked, 'What did you do today?', and replies, 'What did you do today?' Another language difficulty is when the child has a set of phrases that she uses in certain situations which may not mean what is actually said. For example, a child may say she has a sore knee, which to her could mean a pain anywhere in the body (this often occurs in children with autism). It may be better in these situations to use visual cues, such as drawings, photographs, objects or actual props, to back up what the child has said. For example, if the child is talking about a part of the body, have her show you *as well as* tell you, using a drawing, a doll or (if appropriate) her own body. This is also a useful strategy to use for a child who is having word-finding difficulties and is unable to say the word she wants to use. This child may say the wrong word (e.g. leg when she means arm), or describe what she is talking about (e.g. 'You reach out with it'). It may be useful to repeat back to the child what you understand her to have said so that she can correct you if you have misheard or misinterpreted her. Keep in mind, however, that while this may allow for clarification, the child may not be able or willing to correct you.

Finally, a child with an intellectual disability is likely to become tired and overloaded more quickly than the average child of the same age. Some signs of fatigue or overload include becoming stuck on one word or topic; repeating back what you have said (echolalia); a deterioration in the child's speech; or seeming to 'phase out' or simply stopping answering your questions. Other signs include restlessness, yawning or difficulty remaining on the topic. If the child is obviously tired, you should have a break immediately or postpone the interview. It is better to conduct several short interview sessions rather than one long one. It is the quality not quantity of the child's responses that counts. (For further information see Braithwaite & Thompson 2000.)

WHAT ARE AUGMENTATIVE AND ALTERNATIVE COMMUNICATION (AAC) METHODS?

Some children or adolescents with communication impairments may use *augmentative* communication to enhance their speech or *alternative* communication methods to replace their speech. The use of any of these systems does not in any way reflect that the child has a lower intellectual capacity than a child who speaks. In fact, some children who use AAC devices (such as those with physical disabilities like cerebral palsy) have very mild (if any) intellectual disability.

There are two types of AAC systems: electronic and non-electronic. Some of the non-electronic systems include books or boards which contain line drawings, photographs, words, letters or objects which the child points to. Other systems such as signing, natural gesture, facial expression, body language and the child's own idiosyncratic communication are also included in the non-electronic category. The electronic category contains any electronic device which is used for communication. There are a large number of different devices, with different output systems. Some of the devices involve voice output, whereby a message is spoken by the device following activation by the user. Others have outputs such as a paper printout of what has been keyed in by the user. The way a child accesses her device will depend on her physical capabilities. One child may access her device independently, using some part of her body (e.g. her hand) or a piece of apparatus, such as a pointer attached to her head. Another child may require some assistance to access her device, for example, a facilitator who will steady the child's arm or hold the device for her. This is called 'facilitated communication'.

If you are going to interview a child who uses one of these devices, try to find out how the device works before the interview begins. Is it electronic or non-electronic? What is the type of output? How does the child physically use the device (independently or with a facilitator)? These points will allow you to determine how you will position yourself and the child during the interview, and the nature and degree of the communication that is likely to occur. If the child's main form of communication is signing, you should consider using an interpreter. If an interpreter is used who is not familiar with the child, then the interpreter should be given time to build rapport with the child before the interview commences.

If an interview using AAC systems is going to be videotaped, then there are several things to consider. First, before the interview, it is advisable to demonstrate on the video how the device works and how the child uses the device. Second, as always, make sure the camera is placed so that the child can be clearly seen. However, you may also need to check that the output from the device can be clearly heard or seen (as appropriate). If the output cannot be clearly heard or seen, then you may have to repeat or read out was has been said and confirm with the child after each answer that this is what she meant. Third, you need to ascertain before asking the child about body parts whether the child has been taught about them or whether the communication board (if applicable) includes all parts of the body or sexual symbols and words. Some communication boards have been designed specifically for use by child-protection interviewers (Sattler 1998). However, a large number of commonly used boards may have sexual references omitted from them because the child's parents or caregivers see no reason for the child to have access to such words (Westcott & Cross 1996).

Box 4.3   Try this
Tell somebody what you did on the weekend without using any speech. How did this feel? What where the main methods of communication that you used? What did the other person have to do to be able to understand you?

HOW DO I TAILOR AN INTERVIEW TO A CHILD WHO HAS DIFFICULTY HEARING?

Before the interview, find out the nature and degree of the hearing impairment. Next, check out the type of communication difficulty the child may have. Does the child wear hearing aids? Has she got them on? Are they turned on? Do they work? Can the child lip read? Can the child read questions posed in written form? Does the child need a professional interpreter skilled in sign language?

Regardless of the extent of the child's hearing impairment, she is likely to rely somewhat on a combination of lip reading and observation of your non-verbal behaviors. Hence, as always, make sure that you look at the child when addressing her so that she can see your lips and face clearly, and that you speak clearly without mumbling. Also be aware of the room lighting and acoustics. The room should be well lit and free from distracting noises. Adequate light should be reflecting on your face and hands. If there is a strong light behind you, this may obstruct the view of your face.

If an interpreter of sign language is needed, the same principles apply as they do when using an interpreter who speaks another verbal language (see earlier sections in this chapter). In particular, ethical standards require interpreters to sign all speech that would be available to a hearing individual. Hence, you should be careful not to make side comments (e.g. 'I really don't think she is paying attention') to an interpreter in the child's presence (Poole & Lamb 1998).

HOW DO I TAILOR AN INTERVIEW TO A CHILD WHO HAS DIFFICULTY WITH VISION?

As with a child who has a hearing impairment, it is important to establish the nature and extent of any visual impairment before the interview. If the child wears glasses, establish whether she brought them to the interview. If the child has partial vision, make sure you arrange the seating so that the child will be able to see you and any visual cues that you may be using.

Before the interview commences, allow the child time to explore the interview room providing verbal descriptions where needed. Further, spend time establishing the child's understanding of concepts that may be relevant to the interview. Children with visual impairments have a high incidence of language difficulties (Bradley-Johnson 1994; Higgins 1973), but you do not necessarily need to raise your voice to these children (their hearing may be normal). If you wish to use toys and games, make sure they can be adequately used by visually impaired children—colored blocks and drawing tools may be inappropriate. If you are unsure what toys to provide, ask the family or carer what the child's favorite toys are.

Throughout the interview, make sure to inform the child what you are doing at all times (especially if you move position in the room). Unexpected noises (e.g. noises created by recording equipment) can be particularly unnerving if the child cannot see what has caused them. Finally, keep in mind that you may unwittingly use common expressions such as 'Did you *see* the . . .?', which may be meaningless to a child who is blind. If you mistakenly use these expressions, try not to let them embarrass you too much. It is not uncommon for blind people to use them also (Sattler 1998).

HOW DO I ASSESS WHETHER A CHILD IS RESPONDING WITH ANSWERS JUST TO PLEASE ME?

This is an important question to consider when interviewing any child, but it is particularly important when interviewing a child with an intellectual and communication difficulty. While it should never be assumed that children with these backgrounds will be unable to give a reliable interview, they may be more susceptible to leading questions and interviewer's suggestions (Milne & Bull 1996). Response patterns that indicate that bias may be occurring include:

- saying 'don't know' to most questions;
- agreeing with all or most questions (referred to by psychologists as 'affirmation bias' or by some linguists and anthropologists as 'gratuitous concurrence');
- always picking the last or first alternative when presented with forced choice options;
- always answering questions in a socially desirable manner;
- providing stereotypical responses; or
- answering questions impulsively and then recanting the answer.

When such response patterns appear, you may need to provide further confirmation of the information obtained. For example, if the child always responds to a question with 'yes', ask a question for which you know the correct answer to be 'no'. If it appears that the child is merely responding in a way to please you, do not bring this to the attention of the child. It is your responsibility to phrase the questions in a manner that is least likely to result in a biased response from the child (e.g. try using open-ended questions). If this cannot be done, then stop the interview and let the child know you will come back at a later date. In the meantime, ask the child's carers or other professionals who deal with the child how to overcome this problem. Every child has the right to be heard, even if it takes a while to figure out how that can best be achieved.

HOW DO I ASSESS WHETHER A CHILD HAS BEEN COACHED?

A family may be going through a messy divorce and you may have suspicions as to whether the child has been coached by her mother to say she has been abused. How would you check this out?

The interview format remains the same whatever you think is the basis of the allegations of abuse. An open mind and the ability to check alternative hypotheses is still relevant. In fact, the messy divorce merely gives you one more possible hypothesis to check than when interviewing a child whose parents are not divorcing. Further, false allegations are relatively rare. Jones and McGraw (1987) estimated that 2 per cent of child and 6 per cent of adult allegations of child abuse were false (from 576 reports to United States social services). Thoennes and Tjaden (1990) followed a sample of more than 9000 families who were pursuing a custody visitation dispute through the court. Child sexual abuse was alleged in less than 2 per cent of those cases. Of the cases alleging abuse, 33 per cent were viewed as being unlikely to be abuse, 17 per cent were inconclusive and 6 per cent were consciously false, while the remaining cases were considered to be consistent with or likely to be abuse (from 129 cases).

If you suspect that a child has been put up to the allegation, then, as always, interview the child without the parent present and try to get a sense of the context of the allegation. Find out whom the child has spoken to, why Mum brought her here, what Mum has said to the child about the other parent. However, be aware that there is currently no reliable diagnostic test for determining if a child's report is false (Lamb et al. 1997). The use of adult language by the child (e.g. 'I've been molested'), for example, does not mean that the account is fabricated as this information could have been obtained subsequent to a spontaneous disclosure. Behavior that is consistent with a parent's accusations could be the result of 'brainwashing', but some divorces are the result of the abuse allegations, not vice versa. Further, a lack of specific details in a child's account may be because the allegation was made up, but may also be the result of normal developmental or memory limitations (see Chapter 1).

HOW DO I ASSESS RITUAL ABUSE?

The issue of ritual abuse has been highlighted in recent years and interviewers are becoming increasingly concerned about it. However, a suspicion of ritual abuse should not alter your interviewing practice. Alternative hypotheses for the child's behavior or allegation still need to be checked out. Bizarre or illogical statements still need to be followed up or clarified. Details of separate occurrences still need to be obtained. The interview still needs to be child-centered with the child doing as much talking as possible. If you are talking to multiple children, then you need to be particularly careful not to bring up details reported by other children.

If the child has been abused by more than one adult, she may have greater problems than other children in trusting adults, particularly if members of her own family have been involved in the abuse. The child's fears for safety, therefore, may need to be addressed before attempting to interview her.

5

EVALUATING THE PROCESS AND OUTCOME OF AN INTERVIEW

Debriefing is a way of making sense of what has happened during an interview and putting it into perspective. For some, it may involve the expression of fears, worries and concerns to a professional counsellor. For others, it may merely require a discussion of how the interview went with colleagues or professionals who were involved. Debriefing is not only a way of relieving stress. It provides a way of recognizing early signs of burnout and anxiety that may become a problem in the future. It is also important to receive feedback about how you performed in the interview. This chapter examines what happens at the end of an interview and how to debrief and evaluate your performance.

SHOULD I REASSURE A CHILD THAT HE DID THE RIGHT THING TO TELL?

It is important for a child to feel that he has done well to come forward. Always thank the child for talking to you and for his patience and cooperation. However, it is very important that you do not second guess how a child is thinking or feeling. For example, telling a child 'This is not your fault' or 'You are not to blame for this' implies that the child thought it may be his fault. It may not have occurred to him to think about the abuse in this way. On occasions when it is clear that a child blames himself, the comment 'You are not to blame' may set the child thinking 'Why not?', 'But I know I am' or 'How does the interviewer know I'm not to blame . . . I didn't tell her everything'. Indeed, a child who has been abused is unlikely to tell you everything in one interview. Therefore, it is best to leave reassurances or comments about blame to a therapist who is trained in dealing with the child's thoughts and emotions. If *you* are the child's therapist do not confuse information-gathering with therapy. Make note of the child's fears and anxieties regarding blame but address them when you and the child have time on another occasion.

At the end of a disclosure it is important to make sure the child feels he has been listened to and taken seriously whatever he had to say. Whether the child feels this will depend mainly on how you behaved during rather than after the interview. However, just before the child leaves, it is a good idea to engage him for a few minutes in a discussion about something innocuous, light-hearted and unrelated to the abuse. This demonstrates to him that you have no bad feelings about what was said, and may help to put him in a positive mood.

Sometimes following a disclosure a child is concerned about whether the alleged offender will go to jail. Work out a simple answer to this question in advance. You could explain to the child that such decisions are not made by you and they cannot be made immediately. You may need to explain that whether the alleged offender will be charged or sent to jail has little to do with whether the child is believed or not (although it will often seem that way). Do not bring this topic up unless the child does first—it suffers from the same problems associated with 'you are not to blame'. Also, be careful not to make any promises to a child that you cannot keep. If these promises are broken, the child may feel very betrayed.

You may need to explain protective issues to parents and guardians such as how best to keep their child safe. If you are not a child-protection professional, you should contact one immediately and ask her to discuss these matters with the parents. If *you* are the child-protection professional you may need to explain a little about legal processes to the parents. If it is likely that the case will go to court, you could explain how the criminal courts differ in function from the family courts. Further, you could explain what to do should the child continue to talk about the abuse at home. The main point to instruct parents on is that they should not ask the child questions about the abuse unless the child starts talking first. If the child does talk, they should listen and later document what the child says (and the way it was disclosed), as this may help the prosecution case at a later stage.

WHAT DO I SAY TO A CHILD AND PARENT OR GUARDIAN AFTER THE INTERVIEW IS COMPLETED?

When you have completed interviewing a child, your immediate thoughts may be on what *you* need to do next. At this point, however, the needs of the child and parent or guardian should take priority. Make sure you give them time to ask you any questions. They are likely to want to know what happens next. Try to keep them informed as best as you can. You should also tell them you are available if the child or guardian wishes to contact you again. Making the child feel that he can come back at his choosing allows a sense of trust to develop and assists if the child has more to tell at a later time. Providing a business card (for both the child and guardian) ensures that further contact is possible and the invitation is perceived to be genuine.

WHAT WILL DEBRIEFING ACHIEVE?

Debriefing should be useful to achieve two aims. First, to prevent stress affecting you and your job. Second, to allow you to reflect on your performance so that you may improve your skills.

While there are many rewards to working with children, the job can be extremely stressful. Knowing about the harmful ways in which a child was treated can cause distress (only a certain level of 'desensitization' ever occurs). Anger exhibited by families can sometimes be targeted at the interviewer. Pressures of the interview process and dissatisfaction with the outcome of a case can cause a great deal of frustration. However, interviewers often report that the greatest stress factor is the bureaucratic environment in which they work. Common organizational pressures include lack of resources, lack of time, lack of support from supervisors, pressure from other professionals involved in the case, equipment breakdown and frustration with the judicial system (does the phrase 'banging your head against a brick wall' ring a bell?). Many people consider these pressures to be 'just part of the job'. However, they should be taken seriously, as there are times when they can lead to debilitating mental fatigue and breakdown.

Some things you might be able to control or change yourself. Conducting multiple interviews in a single day (when you already have a large caseload) can exacerbate things, and if you strongly identify with a child (e.g. if the child is the same age as your own child) or if you have problems in your personal life (illness, problems with your spouse, financial difficulties, etc.) you might find yourself particularly overwrought. Discussing your work issues can help. If you are a manager or supervisor of a unit, regular discussion groups or informal gatherings with your staff members can help relieve the build-up of stress. Such meetings should provide time for staff to discuss their concerns relating to cases and the organization.

The other benefit of debriefing is that it provides you with the opportunity to reflect on your own performance and to consider ways of improving it. This is most effective if the interview is videotaped so you are not relying on memory (which is unlikely to be 100 per cent accurate). A videotape also allows you to watch and evaluate your non-verbal as well as verbal behaviors. It is important to obtain feedback as close as possible to the interview, in a private setting where confidentiality is maintained. Recording comments and suggestions in a book can be useful as it allows you over time to see how much you have improved!

HOW DO I EVALUATE MY INTERVIEW?

There are three main things to consider when evaluating an interview: the structure of the interview (the sequencing of the questions); the type of questions asked; and the behavioral interaction/rapport between the interviewer and the child. Below is a transcript based on an actual sexual abuse interview. Personal details have been changed (in order to protect the identity of the interviewer and the child). Read through the transcript and evaluate it yourself with the aid of the boxes. Compare your critique with the one at the end.

> I: Hi, my name is Mary. We've got about half an hour together today and I'd like to start by saying to the tape that it's 2.15 p.m. on the 23rd of September 1999. Would you like to tell me your name for the tape too?
> C: Jane.
> I: What is your last name Jane?
> C: Wilson.

I: How old are you?

C: Nine.

I: Do you know when your birthday is?

C: 12th April.

I: Okay. Do you know why you've come here today?

C: Yeah.

I: Now, I think the easiest way of doing this is if you tell me why you think you're here and any questions I need to ask and anything I need to know, I can ask afterwards. Can you tell me why you're here today?

C: Because of what Joe did.

I: Who's Joe?

C: He lives next door.

I: And why have you come here because of Joe?

C: Because he was molesting me.

Box 5.1   Try this

How would you describe the rapport the interviewer has with the child so far? Did the child appear to understand everything the interviewer said? What questions could have been better phrased? Write down how you would have phrased these questions. How well did the interviewer explain the ground rules for the interview?

I: How long have you known Joe?

C: Oh . . . dunno. [Long pause] I think when I was in Mrs Curry's class.

Box 5.2   Try this

What direction is this interview now taking? How well did it follow on from the child saying that Joe was molesting her? What type of questions is the interviewer using here? How could this information have been obtained differently?

I: How did you first get to meet Joe?

C: With Lesley . . . my friend. She took me down there and we were talking and stuff and that's when it happened.

I: So why don't you tell me what happened . . . start at the very beginning . . . and try not to leave anything out.

C: It's just when he started to put his arm around me and started to feel my bum . . . but he's never put his hands down my pants . . . he only done it on Saturday, this once.

I: So he started by putting his arm around you and feeling your bum. Can you tell me more about that?

C: He was trying to get his hand up my T-shirt because I think I had my T-shirt on . . . cause I was wearing a T-shirt under my jumper.

I: And did he manage to get his hand . . .

C: Yeah [child interrupts interviewer mid-sentence].

I: So what was he actually touching?

C: My boobs.

Box 5.3 Try this
What type of questions are now being asked? How is the child responding (i.e. is the child giving more or less information)?

I: What I'm actually trying to get at . . . look, if I touched my foot, I'm touching my tights there, right? . . . I'm touching my shoes there, trousers there and my skin there [points to appropriate parts]. So what was he touching on you?

C: All over.

Box 5.4 Try this
The interviewer uses a demonstration to ask about whether the child was touched on the skin or on top of her clothes. Write down two different ways the interviewer could have sought this information.

I: On your boobs what was he touching?

C: Yeah.

I: He was touching your boobs. What would he be touching . . . was it on top of your clothes?

C: Yeah, at first.

I: At first, then afterwards?

C: Up my T-shirt.

I: Under your T-shirt? [Interviewer appears to mishear child.]
C: Yeah.
I: After he was touching your breast, what happened next?
C: He was on top of me and tried to pull down my clothes. He was forcing himself on me, and I was forcing him off me, but he wouldn't get off.
I: Uh huh. And then?
C: I swore at him and was slapping him and everything . . . punching him and kicking him . . .
I: After he touched you there, where else on your body did he touch you?
C: On my private.
I: What happened?
C: [Child starts crying.]
I: It's all right. You're doing really well. You don't need to get upset, okay? We'll take it slowly, okay?
C: [Child nods . . . long pause.]
I: So let me just go over what you've told me so far and you tell me if I've got anything wrong. When you were in Mrs Curry's class, you went to Joe's house, next door, with your friend Lesley. While you were there, Joe put his arm around you and started to feel you. He put his hand up under your clothes and touched your boobs, and then he tried to pull your clothes off you, and you tried to stop him. After that, he tried to touch you on your private. What happened then?

Box 5.5   Try this
The child did not appear to understand one of the questions asked, and the interviewer did not follow this up. How might the interviewer have clarified the misunderstanding? For the sake of rapport, would it have been better to have ignored this misunderstanding or should the interviewer have checked it out? How do you think the interviewer handled the touching questions? How might these have been worded differently? Was the summary used effectively?

C: He was in the room but I don't think he knew what he was doing. We were playing on the computer and he put his arm around me. We were doing nothing . . .
I: Doing nothing?
C: He just put his arm around me and he moved up close to me

like that [child shuffles in chair] . . . and he was sitting there [child points to other end of couch] and I was sitting here [child points to where she is sitting] and he moved up like that [child shuffles] to move closer to me and put his arm around me and his hand went down my back a bit and I was, like, sitting there.

I: His hand went down your back . . . so what was he touching?

C: Yeah. Just my back there [points to back]. And then he got down closer to my bum and he put his hand down my shorts. He put it down through there and started to feel my bum. I tried to get up and I said, 'Don't!', and I moved away from him.

I: So what was he actually touching?

C: My bum.

I: What part of your bum?

C: This part [child points down between knees].

I: So what was he doing when he was touching there?

C: He was just, like, feeling it . . . feeling my private part.

I: And how did he try to get to your private part?

C: Well, he was, like, just doing that. Trying to get down there but I said, 'Don't', and I moved away onto the floor.

I: Okay. Well, what do you call your private part? Well, obviously you call it your private part. Where is it on you?

C: On the front, down there [child points between legs].

Box 5.6   Try this

What types of questions are being asked and how is the child responding? Is the interviewer following this in a neutral manner and is she exploring alternative hypotheses? Is that appropriate in this case?

I: Did he say anything to you while he was touching your private part?

C: Well, I yelled at him, like, and he goes, 'I was only messing about'.

I: Was there anyone else there while this was happening?

C: My brother was in the kitchen. He came in and he said, 'Were you shouting at him?', and I said, 'Yeah', and he goes, 'Why?', and I go, 'I'll tell you later'. Then I told him what happened.

I: When did you tell him?

C: Well, when I came in and he went back out again, I went back with him and told him what happened.

I: Right. What did your brother say?

C: He just pulled a face and said, 'Dirty idiot'.

I: And did anything else happen that day?

C: No.

I: Can you tell me anything else about what happened . . . any time?

Box 5.7   Try this

Does the interviewer know whether the brother saw any-thing? What else might need to be asked about the brother? What concerns would you have?

C: That's it really.

I: Did you tell your mum?

C: Yeah. On Sunday.

I: And when was the time that your brother was there?

C: It was Saturday that he touched me.

I: When was the time with Lesley? You mentioned Lesley.

C: That was when I first met him.

I: What did he do that time, with Lesley?

C: There were a few times with Lesley. The first one, when I first, like, met him, he just put his arms around me and stuff. Like I said.

I: So how many times has the touching happened?

C: [Child starts to get squeamish and irritated] Lots . . . but I've said everything that he did already.

I: Okay. Can you tell me about Joe, like what he looks like?

C: He's got brown hair, and I think brown eyes.

I: Mmm.

C: And he always wears these horrible grey trousers. And he's got black boots too. And that's all I can say about him. And he smells. Like old boots.

I: What color is his skin?

C: White . . .

I: How old would you say he was?

C: Really old. Like at least 50.

Box 5.8   Try this

There appears to have been multiple occasions when Joe interfered with Jane. How else could this information have been obtained? How did the interviewer's questioning in relation to this matter affect her rapport with the child? Do we know whether Lesley saw anything? How might this be established?

I: Okay. Is there anything else you can think to tell me?

C: I remember going to the shop yesterday and I seen Joe there and he goes 'Hello' to me, and I just went 'Hello' back to act normal.

I: That's the best way to be. Um. Well, let's just go over what you've told me about what Joe did . . . I just want to make sure I've got everything straight. You said Joe put his hand down your bum and touched you on your private part . . . down there [points between legs]. You told your brother, and you told your mum on Sunday. You said that Joe touched you a few times . . . the first time he touched you was when you were in Mrs Curry's class . . . on your boobs. Is that right?

C: Yeah.

I: And the last time he touched you was on Saturday, when he touched you on your private part.

C: Mmm [nods].

I: He's touched you a few times on your boobs when you were with Lesley.

C: Yeah . . . and he did it to Lesley too.

I: And then you told me what he looked like . . . He's got brown hair, maybe brown eyes, grey trousers and black boots, he's about 50 years old and he smells.

C: Like old boots.

I: Is that everything you want to tell me?

C: Yeah.

I: Well, thank you for coming to speak to me about this. Are there any questions you would like to ask me?

C: What are you gonna do to Joe?

I: I don't know. I'm going to have to talk to Lesley, your brother and Joe before I know what might happen.

C: Will he go to jail?

I: I don't know. That's not up to us. Only a judge can decide if somebody goes to jail. I'm afraid we'll have to wait a while until we know what exactly is going to happen, but I promise to let you know as soon as I do. Okay? Remember your mum has my number, and if you remember anything more and you'd like to talk to me later, just ask your mum and she'll bring you here again. Thanks again for coming and talking. You've been a great help. Come with me now and we'll go find your mum.

Box 5.9   Try this
How well did the interviewer conclude the interview? Is there any other information that she could have given the child, or is the conclusion appropriate? Write down what

you would have said. Overall, how good do you think the
interview was? Did the interviewer maintain rapport with
the child? How did the interviewer handle the fluctuations
in rapport? Do you think the child would come back with
more information if she had it?

Overall, we think that the above interview conducted with Jane
is a moderately good interview. The interviewer used many
open-ended questions and obtained a relatively clear account.
However, the account was not clear in terms of the number of
times the alleged offence occurred with Joe, and the specific details
and time of each separate occurrence. As a result, a second
interview appears likely.

In general, the interviewer demonstrated good questioning
skills but she did not always use them in the appropriate place.
She sometimes resorted to closed 'Did you . . .?' and 'Can you
. . .?' questions when open questions could have been used in
their place. Because the interviewer used few leading questions,
she gave the appearance of being neutral and professional. Her
hypothesis for the allegation was broad (i.e. What did Joe do?).
Most of the information was able to be obtained from the child
in a clear manner. However, she might have checked out a number
of additional points that were relevant to the case; for example,
whether the abuse was part of a game, whether digital penetration
was involved and the context of the behavior could have been
further explored.

The child appeared to understand the purpose of the interview
as she disclosed the alleged abuse freely and willingly. However,
the ground rules of the interview could have been better explained
(i.e. instructions to say don't know and to ask the interviewer to
repeat a question if the child did not understand). When the child
did not know the answer to a question, she did not know what
to do (i.e. she said 'Yeah' to a question a number of times that
didn't require a yes/no answer). This could also have been due
to a hearing problem which we assume would have been checked
out prior to the interview.

In general, the interview could have been better handled in
many ways and the interviewer has room for improvement.
However, better questioning is no guarantee that the interviewer
could have obtained more forensically relevant information. The

disclosure of information is up to the child. The interviewer's job is to aid the child to disclose it and support the child to tell it in the most efficient manner. The success is measured by the process, not the outcome of the interview.

Here is a closer critique of the interview.

> I: Hi, my name is Mary. We've got about half an hour together today and I'd like to start by saying to the tape that it's 2.15 p.m. on the 23rd of September 1999. Would you like to tell me your name for the tape too?

Notice she starts saying things for 'the tape'—not a good rapport-building technique as the interviewer is here to talk to the child. She does know the child's name yet asks the child to supply it. Again, this is great for 'the tape' but lousy for rapport. It is more helpful to use the child's name when introducing yourself. Mary doesn't mention her occupation or why she is interviewing the child. Nor does she mention the ground rules for this conversation. A better introduction may have been:

Hi Jane, my name is Mary and I am a social worker. I'd like to talk to you today if that's okay? We have about half an hour to talk about what's been worrying you. Before we get started, there are some things I would like you to know. First, if I ask a question and you don't know what I'm talking about, just tell me. I'll try and explain it better. Second, if I ask you something and you don't know the answer, just say, 'I don't know'. It's important not to guess or make things up. I need to know only what you can remember. If you can't remember, that's fine. Finally, if you need a little break or want a drink or something, again, just tell me. If I can do anything to make you feel more comfortable, just ask and I'll try and help. Okay? Now let's get started . . .

> C: Jane.
> I: What is your last name Jane?
> C: Wilson.
> I: How old are you?
> C: Nine.
> I: Do you know when your birthday is?
> C: 12th April.

All of these questions are closed. None ask the child to talk about anything.

> I: Okay. Do you know why you've come here today?
> C: Yeah.

'Thanks for that' may have been better than 'Okay'. Notice that asking a 'Do you know . . .?' question often results in the child giving only a yes or no answer and then another question needs to be asked. Again, this is not helpful when trying to encourage a child to talk.

> I: Now, I think the easiest way of doing this is if you tell me why you think you're here and any questions I need to ask and anything I need to know, I can ask afterwards. Can you tell me why you're here today?

The child has obviously told someone something already and knows why she is here. That makes your job easier. Notice the 'I think the easiest way of doing this' implies that this is not going to be easy. That sentence is also very long. It may have been helpful to break it up more.

> C: Because of what Joe did.
> I: Who's Joe?

The child wants to talk about what Joe did. A better response would have been to repeat the last part of the sentence as a question: '. . . What Joe did?' You can find out who Joe is later.

> C: He lives next door.
> I: And why have you come here because of Joe?

An odd phrase. Why not 'And what did Joe do?'

> C: Because he was molesting me.
> I: How long have you known Joe?

The term 'molesting' seems a little old for this nine-year-old child. Asking the child about that may have been useful in determining whether she fully understood its meaning, for example, by gently repeating the last part of her sentence back as a question, '. . . Molesting you?' How long she has known Joe seems irrelevant at this point.

> C: Oh . . . dunno. [Long pause] I think when I was in Mrs Curry's class.
> I: How did you first get to meet Joe?

Notice the interviewer doesn't pick up on the conversation flow about Mrs Curry's class, that is, she could have asked, 'When were you in Mrs Curry's class?' or, better still, 'Tell me about being in Mrs Curry's class'.

C: With Lesley . . . my friend. She took me down there and we were talking and stuff and that's when it happened.
I: So why don't you tell me what happened . . . start at the very beginning . . . and try not to leave anything out.

The interviewer tries to introduce a ground rule. However, it sits awkwardly here. Gently asking 'What happened?' would have been fine.

C: It's just when he started to put his arm around me and started to feel my bum . . . but he's never put his hands down my pants . . . he only done it on Saturday, this once.
I: So he started by putting his arm around you and feeling your bum. Can you tell me more about that?

'Can you' questions are usually answered with 'yes' or 'no' by a young child. Instead, try gently saying, 'Tell me more about that'.

C: He was trying to get his hand up my T-shirt because I think I had my T-shirt on . . . cause I was wearing a T-shirt under my jumper.
I: And did he manage to get his hand . . .

Notice that the previous open question gets a far better response from the child than this yes/no closed question . . .

C: Yeah [child interrupts interviewer mid-sentence].
I: So what was he actually touching?

The interviewer is seeking clarification, but it may be a little early to do that. Asking 'What happened next?' might have been more effective in keeping the child talking.

C: My boobs.
I: What I'm actually trying to get at . . . look, if I touched my foot, I'm touching my tights there, right? . . . I'm touching my shoes there, trousers there and my skin there [points to appropriate parts]. So what was he touching on you?

A concrete example can be helpful when you're not sure how to explain things . . .

C: All over.

Not that it always works!

I: On your boobs what was he touching?
C: Yeah.
I: He was touching your boobs. What would he be touching . . . was it on top of your clothes?

102

Notice the child has said she was being touched 'all over' and when the interviewer directs the attention back to the child's 'boobs', the child is asked where she was touched on the boobs. However, nowhere in this question is a sequence of events clarified. That is, what about asking, 'Let's start at the beginning and go through exactly what happened . . .'

C: Yeah, at first.
I: At first, then afterwards?

We have come back to the sequence of events thanks to the child.

C: Up my T-shirt.
I: Under your T-shirt? [Interviewer appears to mishear child.]
C: Yeah.

Yes, the interviewer misheard the child but notice that the child didn't correct her. Perhaps this is because 'up' and 'under' in this situation meant the same thing.

I: After he was touching your breast, what happened next?

A good open question.

C: He was on top of me and tried to pull down my clothes. He was forcing himself on me, and I was forcing him off me, but he wouldn't get off.
I: Uh huh. And then?

Excellent. Notice how the interviewer is doing less talking and, as a result, the child is now doing a lot more talking.

C: I swore at him and was slapping him and everything . . . punching him and kicking him . . .
I: After he touched you there, where else on your body did he touch you?

Notice how the child is talking about her reaction—she is trying to say that she tried to stop him. Sometimes this may be exaggerated to stress that the child tried everything in her power to prevent the abuse happening. The interviewer recognizes this and decides to ignore this statement by the child. However, the interviewer may have enhanced the rapport with the child by acknowledging this behavior (i.e. 'You tried to stop him . . . and after he touched you there . . .').

C: On my private.
I: What happened?
C: [Child starts crying.]

103

I: It's all right. You're doing really well. You don't need to get upset, okay? We'll take it slowly, okay?

The interviewer is trying hard to comfort the child. 'You don't need to get upset, okay' is a common phrase but not a useful one in this context. Try 'Would you like a couple of minutes break?', or instead offer the child tissues or a drink of water. Merely sitting with the child quietly while she gains composure is better than talking to her. She actually might not want to stop talking.

C: [Child nods . . . long pause.]
I: So let me just go over what you've told me so far and you tell me if I've got anything wrong. When you were in Mrs Curry's class, you went to Joe's house, next door, with your friend Lesley. While you were there, Joe put his arm around you and started to feel you. He put his hand up under your clothes and touched your boobs, and then he tried to pull your clothes off you, and you tried to stop him. After that, he tried to touch you on your private. What happened then?

Good re-introduction. While revising everything the child says is not necessary, it can help the interviewer and child get straight in their minds exactly what has been said so far. Revising also offers the child the opportunity to correct the interviewer. This ground rule was clearly explained here.

C: He was in the room but I don't think he knew what he was doing. We were playing on the computer and he put his arm around me. We were doing nothing . . .
I: Doing nothing?

This question worked fine but may sound like an accusation. Try 'Then what happened?'

C: He just put his arm around me and he moved up close to me like that [child shuffles in chair] . . . and he was sitting there [child points to other end of couch] and I was sitting here [child points to where she is sitting] and he moved up like that [child shuffles] to move closer to me and put his arm around me and his hand went down my back a bit and I was, like, sitting there.
I: His hand went down your back . . . so what was he touching?
C: Yeah. Just my back there [points to back]. And then he got down closer to my bum and he put his hand down my shorts. He put it down through there and started to feel my bum. I tried to get up and I said, 'Don't!', and I moved away from him.
I: So what was he actually touching?

Notice that the child wants to keep talking about what happened and the interviewer wants to know specifically what has been touched. It's always best to let the child say what she wants first. The interviewer can return later and clarify what was actually touched.

> C: My bum.
> I: What part of your bum?
> C: This part [child points down between knees].
> I: So what was he doing when he was touching there?
> C: He was just, like, feeling it . . . feeling my private part.
> I: And how did he try to get to your private part?

These are specific questions that generally result in higher error rates. But they are needed here to clarify exactly what was happening.

> C: Well, he was, like, just doing that. Trying to get down there but I said, 'Don't', and I moved away onto the floor.
> I: Okay. Well, what do you call your private part? Well, obviously you call it your private part. Where is it on you?

Again the child is trying to say she tried to stop Joe, and again the interviewer ignores it. Try not to ignore it. Say something like, 'So you moved away [pause] . . . What do you call. . .?' By repeating the words of the child you are letting the child know that you are listening and understand what she is saying.

> C: On the front, down there [child points between legs].
> I: Did he say anything to you while he was touching your private part?
> C: Well, I yelled at him, like, and he goes, 'I was only messing about'.
> I: Was there anyone else there while this was happening?

Again the interviewer ignores the child's attempts at getting Joe to stop . . .

> C: My brother was in the kitchen. He came in and he said, 'Were you shouting at him?', and I said, 'Yeah', and he goes, 'Why?', and I go, 'I'll tell you later'. Then I told him what happened.
> I: When did you tell him?

'What did you tell him?' may have been a better question.

> C: Well, when I came in and he went back out again, I went back with him and told him what happened.
> I: Right. What did your brother say?
> C: He just pulled a face and said, 'Dirty idiot'.
> I: And did anything else happen that day?

C: No.
I: Can you tell me anything else about what happened . . . any time?
C: That's it really.
I: Did you tell your mum?

'Did you tell anyone else?' may have been more useful.

C: Yeah. On Sunday.
I: And when was the time that your brother was there?
C: It was Saturday that he touched me.
I: When was the time with Lesley? You mentioned Lesley.
C: That was when I first met him.
I: What did he do that time, with Lesley?
C: There were a few times with Lesley. The first one, when I first, like, met him, he just put his arms around me and stuff. Like I said.
I: So how many times has the touching happened?
C: [Child starts to get squeamish and irritated] Lots . . . but I've said everything that he did already.
I: Okay. Can you tell me about Joe, like what he looks like?

The interviewer asked a few questions to clarify things and the child obviously didn't want to talk about what happened any more. It is a good idea to explain why the specific details are needed.

C: He's got brown hair, and I think brown eyes.
I: Mmm.
C: And he always wears these horrible grey trousers. And he's got black boots too. And that's all I can say about him. And he smells. Like old boots
I: What color is his skin?
C: White . . .
I: How old would you say he was?
C: Really old. Like at least 50.

Here the interviewer could have used herself as a reference point, for example, 'Is he younger or older than me?'

I: Okay. Is there anything else you can think to tell me?
C: I remember going to the shop yesterday and I seen Joe there and he goes 'Hello' to me, and I just went 'Hello' back to act normal.
I: That's the best way to be. Um. Well, let's just go over what you've told me about what Joe did . . . I just want to make sure I've got everything straight. You said Joe put his hand down your bum and touched you on your private part . . . down there [points between legs]. You told your brother, and you told your mum on Sunday. You said that Joe touched you a few times . . . the first time he touched you was when you were in Mrs Curry's class . . . on your boobs. Is that right?
C: Yeah.

I: And the last time he touched you was on Saturday, when he touched you on your private part.
C: Mmm [nods].
I: He's touched you a few times on your boobs when you were with Lesley.
C: Yeah . . . and he did it to Lesley too.
I: And then you told me what he looked like . . . He's got brown hair, maybe brown eyes, grey trousers and black boots, he's about 50 years old and he smells.
C: Like old boots.

Good summary. It was also good to see the child play an active role in the revision phase. The interviewer encouraged this.

I: Is that everything you want to tell me?
C: Yeah.

Again, closed questions lead to closed answers.

I: Well, thank you for coming to speak to me about this. Are there any questions you would like to ask me?

Good question. The interviewer immediately focused on the child's needs.

C: What are you gonna do to Joe?
I: I don't know. I'm going to have to talk to Lesley, your brother and Joe before I know what might happen.

Good answer.

C: Will he go to jail?
I: I don't know. That's not up to us. Only a judge can decide if somebody goes to jail. I'm afraid we'll have to wait a while until we know what exactly is going to happen, but I promise to let you know as soon as I do. Okay? Remember your mum has my number, and if you remember anything more and you'd like to talk to me later, just ask your mum and she'll bring you here again. Thanks again for coming and talking. You've been a great help. Come with me now and we'll go find your mum.

Good closure. The interviewer was honest and sincere and didn't make any false promises that she could not keep.

Box 5.10   Try this
Obtain an interview that either you or a colleague conducted.

A videotape or audiotape is preferable, but a transcript will do. Answer the following questions about the interview.

- What aspects of the interview went well?
- What areas could be improved on? Give examples.
- What questioning techniques worked in obtaining free narrative from the child? Which questions hindered the child-centered process?
- How well was the interviewer able to establish rapport with the interviewee? Does the rapport-building meet the interview's purpose (i.e. to get the child talking as much as possible)?
- Was the interviewer objective, neutral (i.e. did she explore alternative hypotheses)? How can you tell?
- Did the interviewer obtain the necessary details or elements of the offence?
- Did the interviewer adapt her style to the developmental level of the child and the child's emotional needs? Give examples.
- How did the interviewer conclude the interview?

WHAT IS STATEMENT VALIDITY ANALYSIS?

Statement Validity Analysis (SVA) and Criterion Based Content Analysis (CBCA) are both methods of evaluating the truthfulness of the child's report rather than the appropriateness of your interviewing technique. They both require that the questions asked are well phrased and mainly open-ended and that the child reports a lot of detail. However, the reliability of these methods in proving the validity of a child's interviews about sexual assault has been seriously questioned. It is therefore advisable not to use either system until more research has been done. (See Lamb et al. 1997 for a review of CBCA.)

HOW DO I GIVE FEEDBACK TO A TEAM OF INTERVIEWERS?

When providing feedback to others about their performance, it is important to make them feel good about your opinions and thus receive them more easily. There are a few tips you could use that may help.

First, try to create a relaxed atmosphere. Tea, coffee and biscuits can do wonders. Choose a time in the day when you will not be interrupted and you can both relax. First thing in the morning can be a very good time.

Second, allow your colleague to comment on how he thinks he performed in the interview before making your comments. Interviewers often recognize their mistakes in hindsight and may be able to generate alternative responses. This also provides you with an insight into the nature of the interviewer's problems (e.g. acquiring knowledge of correct strategies, or putting the knowledge into practice). Make sure you don't sit and nod at all the claimed errors—if the interviewer is being too hard on himself, say so.

Third, when providing your feedback, start with what aspects of the interview you think worked well. If the positive aspects are heard first, the negative aspects are more likely to be listened to. When describing a negative aspect, try to be as specific as possible in pinpointing what the interviewer did wrong (i.e. provide examples). Then state how to improve the performance. For example, instead of saying, 'You were very leading', you might say, 'Five of the first ten questions in the interview were about the alleged perpetrator. Letting the child talk about what happened first may be more helpful. That way we would be certain that he (the alleged perpetrator) was the one and only person we need to be investigating.'

Fourth, when providing alternative interviewing strategies, try to work as a team. If you generate suggestions together, it is much more empowering for the interviewer, and he will be more likely to remember and take on any solutions or suggestions in future. It may be useful to offer time (if needed) for the interviewer to practise alternative behaviors and questioning styles in role plays. Repeated practise via role plays or 'refresher' training activities is essential for improving interviewing skills (Fisher 1995), and through role plays the interviewer comes to feel more in control once new skills are obtained.

Finally, it is important to review an interview gently. Choose just two or three of the main problems to criticize each time you review a tape. The person is not likely to want to make improvements if he feels attacked or his confidence is totally depleted. It is important to work together, and to draw on the experience and expertise of all members of the team in which you work.

Appendix 3 sets out a form for use in examining either your own videotape or that of others. You may like to adapt it to suit your own purposes.

HOW DO I DEAL WITH MY ANGER WHEN I AM EVALUATED?

If you are feeling insecure about your interviewing skills, you will find it more difficult to handle feedback. The best idea is to relax. You are learning to interview—even the best interviewers are always learning. Know that there will be times when you fail. Everyone does. Failure is part of learning. Expert interviewers tend to be those people who are eager to learn about and implement suggestions for improving their performance. So seek out the feedback (ask for it if you don't get it), and try to make the most of it to improve your performance.

There will also be times when you feel your interviewing skills are superior to your supervisor's. This can result in resentment at being criticized by someone with inferior skills. Try to listen to the criticism by your supervisor rather than argue with him. It is merely an opinion, and everyone is entitled to that. Make sure that you fully understand what is being said, though, so you can judge whether the criticism is just.

HOW DO I PUT THE COMMENTS FROM MY EVALUATION INTO PRACTISE?

Knowing how to conduct a good interview does not mean that you have the skills to put that knowledge into practice (Stevenson, Leung & Cheung 1992). Indeed, some of the most prominent researchers and experts in the area of children's testimony openly admit that they would not be good interviewers. 'On the job' you have many things to attend to at the same time: colleagues may be communicating with you from another room; you may be trying to think about possible avenues or leads to follow; and you will be trying to engage the child, listen to his account and take notes as well. In pressured situations like this, it is your best learned skills that are going to be on the 'tip of your tongue'. You will not have the time to ponder or practice alternative ways of

110

phrasing a question. Thus the importance of feedback and role play.

Finally, experience without critical feedback can also be to your disadvantage if it creates 'bad habits' that may be difficult to break in the future. Ongoing practise with critical feedback is the only way to ensure that you are getting the right experience needed to obtain the most accurate and detailed report from the child.

APPENDIX 1: SUGGESTED SOLUTIONS TO BOXES

CHAPTER 1   UNDERSTANDING A CHILD'S MIND

Box 1.2

A child who was sexually assaulted but previously knew nothing about sex would find it more difficult to remember and explain what happened during the assault compared to a child who had been sexually assaulted numerous times. When a child is assaulted repeatedly, she begins to develop a picture of what generally occurs on these occasions (i.e. the sequence of actions and how these actions differ from other non-abusive experiences). This general picture or framework about what usually happens during the abuse is very useful in helping the child to remember or 'reconstruct' what was likely to have happened one of the times.

However, a child who has been abused multiple times would find it difficult to remember *exactly* what happened one time as opposed to other similar times she was assaulted. Remembering details that were particular to one of the instances (i.e. what the offender was wearing, what he did and said, and where other people were) is a very difficult task, as children (like adults) confuse the various instances in memory. Children who were abused only once don't have this problem of trying to separate one instance from other instances. Hence, if the interview requires the child to remember numerous specific details about a *particular time* on which the child was assaulted (as opposed to what generally occurs), the task of remembering would probably be easier for the child who experienced the abuse only once.

Box 1.4

The main way to find out what phrases a child uses for various parts of her body is to ask the child to point to these parts on her own body. It may be better to do this than to ask her to label a drawing or picture, because it helps the child realize that you are talking about her body. It is best to start naming the body parts at the head, eyes, nose, ears, chin, mouth, shoulders and then to move down the body. Do not focus unduly on the sexual body parts or finish the questioning on these parts. Instead, it is better to continue (after identifying these sexual parts) all the way down to the child's knees, ankles and toes. It may also be helpful if you point to the relevant parts on your own body while the child points to them on hers, so the young child can mimic what you are doing and not get confused.

The interview below is an example of the format that could be taken, which combines asking about the names for body parts with finding out about possible injuries to that body part:

> What is this part of the body called? [Interviewer points to head.]
> Has anyone ever hurt you on top of your head?
> Tell me what happened when your head was hurt.
> What is this part of the body called? [Interviewer points to eyes.]
> Has anyone ever hurt your eyes?
> Tell me what happened when your eyes were hurt.
> What is this part of the body called? [Interviewer points to nose.]
> Has anyone ever hurt your nose?
> Tell me what happened when your nose was hurt.
> What is this part of the body called? [Interviewer points to mouth.]
> Has anyone ever hurt your mouth?
> Tell me what happened when your mouth was hurt.
> What is this part of the body called? [Interviewer points to shoulders.]
> Has anyone ever hurt your shoulders?
> Tell me what happened when your shoulders were hurt.
> What is this part of the body called? [Interviewer points to arms.]
> Has anyone ever hurt your arms?
> Tell me what happened when your arms were hurt.
> What is this part of the body called? [Interviewer points to hands.]
> Has anyone ever hurt your hands?
> Tell me what happened when your hands were hurt.
> What is this part of the body called? [Interviewer points to chest.]

Has anyone ever hurt your chest?
Tell me what happened when your chest was hurt.
What is this part of the body called? [Interviewer points to tummy.]
Has anyone ever hurt your tummy?
Tell me what happened when your tummy was hurt.
What is this part of the body called? [Interviewer points to bottom.]
Has anyone ever hurt your bottom?
Tell me what happened when your bottom was hurt.
What is this part of the body called? [Interviewer points to penis/vulva.]
Has anyone ever hurt your front bottom?
Tell me what happened when your front bottom was hurt.
What is this part of the body called? [Interviewer points to legs.]
Has anyone ever hurt your legs?
Tell me what happened when your legs were hurt.
What is this part of the body called? [Interviewer points to feet.]
Has anyone ever hurt your feet?
Tell me what happened when your feet were hurt.

It is worth noting that often children will report all their aches and pains as they do not know specifically what information is being sought. This is a great opportunity not only to check specific injuries you want to know about but also to find out what other injuries the child has had. Such stories of past injuries often build rapport as most children love telling the gruesome details of their many battles.

This interview technique is used in the systematic approach to gathering evidence (see Roberts & Glasgow 1993 for more information).

To learn more about the child's knowledge of sexual acts, it is best to ask a child open-ended questions such as, 'What happened first?', 'What happened then?' The questions should be simply phrased, using words that the child understands, and using the subject-verb-object format where possible. For example, if the child says that Joe did something bad to her, it would be better to ask 'What did Joe do to you?' as opposed to 'What happened to you?'

Box 1.5

Generally, it is very difficult for a parent to coach a child to actually *believe* a false allegation. However, some techniques a parent could use are mentioned in Table 1.2. The parent could imply that the abuse had happened a while ago, and that surely the child remembers it because everyone knows it is true. She could tell the child what, where and how the abuse happened so that the child starts to get a picture of what abuse means and what allegedly happened to her. She could ask leading questions (that include details about the fictitious abuse), she could give the child rewards for talking about it, and could punish the child when she denies that anything happened. Even subtle punishments like withdrawing affection or privileges are likely to work. (For more information, see Chapter 4 'How do I assess whether a child has been coached?') It is important to note, however, that a parent would find it easier to coach a preschool child into believing that her other parent had abused her than a school-aged child, as younger children are more suggestible.

For a child to make up an allegation of sexual abuse on her own (without prompting from an adult), she would need to know something about what sex is and how it is done. She would also need to know that sex with an adult is wrong and that certain consequences may follow from a disclosure of sexual abuse with an adult (i.e. that if she accuses someone of it, they might get into trouble from the police). In addition, she would need good deception skills, and the ability to remain consistent in her story over time. A child usually doesn't have these abilities until her teens.

Box 1.6

Children differ greatly in their emotional responses to telling a secret or lying to keep it. Some think that telling a secret is bad and lying to keep the secret is not really lying, it's keeping the secret. Other children tell the secret because they are scared to keep it. It is important to recognize the 'catch 22' situation that children may see themselves in. That is, they're damned if they do tell (for being a 'tell-tale') and they're damned if they don't (for being a liar to keep the secret, or being held partly guilty for the crime as they did not report it).

Box 1.7

Phrase	Alternative
Tell me about that in more detail . . .	Tell me more about the time in the bathroom . . .
I'd just like to pause the camera while . . .	I'll just turn the camera off while . . .
Are you aware that . . .	Do you know that . . .

(cont.)

Phrase	Alternative
Can you describe the man . . .	Tell me what the man looked like . . .
Can you clarify whether . . .	Tell me more about . . .
You said earlier . . .	Before, you said . . .
In reference to . . .	About the . . .
Your mother alleged that . . .	Your mother said that . . .
State your name . . .	Tell me your name . . .
Speak about the matter concerning David . . .	Talk about what happened with David . . .
Subsequently . . .	After that . . .
I'd like to ascertain . . .	I'd like to work out . . .
In regard to the bathroom incident . . .	About the time in the bathroom . . .
At approximately . . .	About . . .
I put it to you that it was later . . .	Maybe it was later . . .
When did it commence . . .	When did it begin . . .
Can you clarify . . .	Explain more about . . .
Please indicate . . .	Please tell me . . .
I know it is difficult to explain . . .	I know it is hard to talk about . . .
Suspect . . .	Person who may have done something wrong . . .
In sequence . . .	In the right order . . .
Please elaborate . . .	Please tell me more about . . .
Talk me through the incident . . .	Tell me what happened . . .
Observe how I . . .	Watch how I . . .
What is your current address?	Where do you live?
Report . . .	Tell me . . .
Take a written statement . . .	Write down everything you tell me . . .
Matter . . .	What happened . . .
Acknowledge . . .	Agree . . .
Now I'd like to review . . .	Let's go over . . .
Witnessed . . .	Saw . . .
The occasion of . . .	The time when . . .
Tell me the facts . . .	Tell me only what actually happened . . .
His age . . .	How old he is . . .
Did you hear the conversation . . .	Did you hear what Joe and Matt were saying . . .
Let me rephrase that . . .	Let me say that another way . . .
View this photograph . . .	Look at this picture . . .
Prior to his arrival . . .	Before he came in . . .

CHAPTER 2   PREPARATION AND PLANNING OF THE INTERVIEW

Box 2.2

These are just suggestions and should be modified according to your needs.

Consent information for parent/guardian
We [SPECIFY NAME] wish to interview your child. We would also like to videotape that interview. [USE FOLLOWING IF APPROPRIATE] It is now possible for a videotaped interview with a child to be played in court if there are legal proceedings.

The videotaped interview will be kept under lock and key and access will be restricted to those needing it for the legal proceedings.

At times videotaped interviews are viewed by observers in order to evaluate interview procedures. The interviewing team evaluates only the interviewers. This evaluation will not interfere with your child's case in any way. The aim of the evaluation is to feed back information about good practice and successful interviewing techniques. This will help other children who are interviewed and ensure that the videotaped interviews are acceptable to the courts.

We would be grateful if you would sign the attached form to show that you have read the above and that you give your consent to the videotape of the interview.

You may withdraw your consent for the video to be viewed at any time you wish.

Consent information form for interviewees
You are about to be interviewed. We [insert names or organisation] would like to know whether we could videotape your interview. The videotape is helpful for the interviewer and can be shown in court.

The videotape is also helpful in showing us whether the people who interview you are doing a good job by asking you the right questions. If you don't want us to check out the questions by looking at your tape, we won't.

If you would like us to look at the tape, please write your name on the next page. If you're not sure, that's fine, we won't look at the tape.

Thanks very much.

Consent form for parent/guardian
I have read and understood the relevant consent information form.
Interviewee: _____
Parent/Guardian: _____
Date: _____
Please tick one of the following:
[ ] I agree [ ] I do not agree
that *(interviewee)* can be videotaped during the interview.
Signed: _____
Printed name: _____
Date: _____
If you have any further questions or concerns, please contact *(interviewer)* on *(phone)*, *(fax)* or by email on *(email address)*.

Consent form for interviewee
I have read the information.
Interviewee: _____
Date: _____
Please tick one of the following:
[ ] Yes, I am happy to be videotaped
[ ] No, I do not want to be videotaped
Please tick one of the following:
[ ] I do not want people looking at my tape
[ ] People can look at my tape
Signed: _____
Printed name: _____
Date: _____

Box 2.4

The information you need to obtain before organizing an interview time and place for the child is:

- the hospital routine;
- when the child eats;
- when medication, especially pain medication, is given;

118

- when the child is most alert;
- when the child's family normally comes to visit.

Often the best time to interview a child in hospital is mid-morning. The child is usually awake, has eaten, is comfortable, and it's usually before any visitors (e.g. family) have arrived. However, every child is different as is his treatment routine.

The ward may not be the best place to conduct an interview. It may seem convenient but it can be very distracting for the child, especially if there are several children in the ward. It can also be very embarrassing to talk about highly personal incidents around other people. It is best to find a place outside the ward. You may find that the child appreciates this time away. What needs to be considered, however, is the availability of quality space—a cupboard-sized room with no windows is not recommended. If the child has mobility problems, the bigger the interview room the better. If a room is unavailable, consider going outside into quiet, private gardens, if they are available (but remember this limits the possibility of videotaping).

Box 2.5

In a discussion between a child and his teacher about a science project, it is generally accepted that the teacher knows more about the topic than the child. The whole purpose of the project (which is usually constructed by the teacher) is for the child to learn about the topic. Therefore, if the child is on the wrong track or gets an answer wrong, the teacher would generally tell the child this and in some cases correct the answer. At other times, the teacher may not tell the child the answer but repeat the question or task and let the child have another go at trying to answer it. It is generally acceptable, therefore, for the child to make mistakes and to guess an answer. This tells the teacher that the child is involved in the task and is actively trying to get it right, and it gives the teacher some idea of where the child may be going wrong. There is no harm in getting an answer wrong. The teacher knows the answer and will make sure the child eventually gets it right.

Teachers are not generally interested in knowing precisely where or how a child learned something. It could have come from a variety of sources—books, television programs, radio shows or previous lessons at school. Such sources may be hard for the child to identify.

The ground rules described above are very different from the

119

ground rules of an interview where the goal is to obtain accurate information from a child about a life experience (i.e. an injury or abusive event) that you know little, or nothing, about. This means that you cannot accurately correct the child. It is important, therefore, to make sure that when you are interviewing a child for this purpose the ground rules outlined in Table 2.3 are clearly explained. Otherwise, the child may misunderstand what it is he is supposed to do and say in the interview.

Box 2.6

In the pre-interview for the child in hospital you should assess:

- how comprehendable the child's language is (if the child is heavily medicated, for example, this may slur his speech);
- whether other assistance in communication is needed (e.g. an interpreter or drawing utensils);
- the child's attention span and concentration—a child having chemotherapy may have good concentration but this may be interrupted by surges of nausea;
- whether the medical condition allows the child to be interviewed;
- whether it would be better to have multiple short sessions or one relatively long session.

You would explain the interview process and the ground rules in the same way as you would explain the interview to a child who is not in hospital. However, you may need to emphasize that if the child gets too tired or feels sick at any time during the interview, he should tell you this so that you can stop the interview and let him get some rest.

Deciding which toys you should take to the interview is difficult. You must watch that you are not patronizing the child and that the toys are not seen as a bribe for talking to the interviewer. For example, a video game may be seen as a gift to the child for speaking to you. A good toy to take along is drawing equipment because it could be useful for communication.

CHAPTER 3   ESSENTIAL ELEMENTS OF THE INTERVIEW

Box 3.3

Hi Jane, my name is Mary and I am a social worker. I'd like to talk to you today if that's okay? We have about half an hour together today. Before we get started, there are some things I would like you to know. First, if I ask a question and you don't know what I'm talking about, just tell me. I'll try and explain it better. Second, if I ask you something and you don't know the answer, just say 'I don't know'. It's important not to guess or make things up. I need to know only what you can remember. Tell me everything you remember, even the little things that you don't think are important. If you can't remember, that's fine. I will not get angry or upset with you. Also, this interview is going to be videotaped. Is that okay? Having a videotape of the interview helps me to look over all the things we have talked about. Finally, if you need a little break or want a drink or something, just tell me. If I can do anything to make you feel more comfortable, just ask and I'll try and help. Okay? Now let's get started . . .

Box 3.6

You might ask Sarah and Mikey what normally happens when Katherine and Tom babysit. You would make the questions simpler for Mikey but you would still use open-ended questions such as, 'Tell me what usually happens when Katherine and Tom come over to visit'. Further, Mikey is likely to need more time, prompts and non-verbal encouragers to help him talk (see Chapter 3 'How do I keep a young child talking?').

Once the child starts talking about the abuse, it is useful to obtain details regarding what happened, who did it, where the children were when it happened, and if anyone else saw or heard the above. This is outlined in Table 3.4.

CHAPTER 4   TAILORING THE INTERVIEW TO THE CHILD'S NEEDS

Box 4.2

Hello, my name is Mary. I am a psychologist. My job is to listen to problems children are having. What is your name? Today, I would like to talk to you for about half an hour. Is that okay? I'm going to ask you some questions. If you don't understand a question, let me know and I'll try and say it differently. If you don't know the answer, you can say 'I don't know'.

In a situation where you are interviewing an emotionally disturbed child, take note of the seating arrangements. Do not have any toys available that may be used as projectiles or could be used to injure the child or yourself. Use eye contact to encourage the child but be careful not to stare, as this is likely to unsettle the child. The best time to start with the interview is when the child is calm and relaxed, and you should try to have a calm and relaxed demeanour yourself.

APPENDIX 2: REFERENCES FOR INTERVIEWING DIFFERENT CULTURAL GROUPS

The following references are good starting points when considering issues of culture.

GENERAL

Palmer, S. & Laungani, P. (eds) 1999, *Counselling in a Multicultural Society*, Sage Publications, London.

Phillips, M. 1993, 'Investigative interviewing: issues of race and culture' in *Investigative Interviewing with Children: Trainers Pack*, Open University, Milton Keynes.

Ponterotto, J., Casas, J., Suzuki, L. & Alexander, C. (eds), 1995 *Handbook of Multicultural Counselling*, Sage Publications, Thousands Oaks, CA.

SPECIFIC

Cole, E. 1998, 'Immigrant and refugee children: Challenges and opportunities for education and mental health services', *Canadian Journal of School Psychology*, vol. 14, pp. 36–50.

Dimigen, G. 1993, 'Second language learning by children of Asian descent in Great Britain', *Psychologia: an International Journal of Psychology in the Orient*, vol. 35, pp. 96–100.

Eslea, M. & Mukhtar, K. 2000, 'Bullying and racism among Asian schoolchildren in Britain', *Educational Research*, vol. 42, pp. 207–217.

Gupta, A. 1997, 'Black children and the Memorandum', *Perspectives on the Memorandum: Policy, practice and research in investigative interviewing* eds H. Westcott & J. Jones, Arena, Aldershot, England, pp. 81–93.

Powell, M. B. in press, 'P.R.I.D.E.: The essential elements of a forenisc interview with an Aboriginal person', *Australian Psychologist.*

APPENDIX 3: SELF-ASSESSMENT FORM

1. Code number: _____   5. Number of interviewers: __
2. Date of interview: _____   6. Main interviewer: _____
3. Age of child: _____   7. Length of interview:_____
4. Sex of child: F/M _____

TECHNICAL ASPECTS OF THE INTERVIEW

8. The room is: a Clinical
                 b Comfortable
                 c Child-Centered

The child had available:
 9. Y/N   Food
10. Y/N   Drink
11. Y/N   Drawing materials
12. Y/N   Toys/blocks
13. Y/N   Models (representational)
14. Y/N   Normal dolls
15. Y/N   Anatomical dolls

16. Characteristics of the child throughout the interview:
a Easily distracted b Hyperactive c Defensive d Eager to please
e Distressed f Articulate g Inarticulate h Task-focused
i Withdrawn j Calm

125

RAPPORT

17. Length of rapport: _____

Verbal aspects

Interviewer:
18. Y/N   Introduces self and/or explains job
19. Y/N   Mentions the reason for interview
20. Y/N   Points out cameras to child (if used)
21. Y/N   Explains importance of telling the truth
22. Y/N   Asks child the difference between truth and a lie
23. Y/N   Mentions acceptability of saying 'I don't know'
24. Y/N   Mentions 'ground rules' (e.g. allowed to use any words)

Questions included:
25. Y/N   Appropriate vocabulary
26. Y/N   Simple sentences
27. Y/N   Pauses for child to speak uninterrupted
28. Y/N   Rapport is established
29. Y/N   Rapport connects into the main interview

Non-verbal aspects

30. Y/N   Child's speech fluent   33. Y/N   Interviewer's speech fluent

31. Y/N   Child is relaxed   34. Y/N   Interviewer is relaxed
32. Y/N   Child holds eye contact   35. Y/N   Interviewer holds eye contact

FREE NARRATIVE ACCOUNT

36. Length of free narrative: _____

Verbal aspects

Interviewer:
37. Y/N   Uses 'wide' opening phrases
38. Y/N   Allows child to speak uninterrupted
39. Y/N   Allows for pauses in conversation
40. Y/N   Uses short verbal noises (e.g. ah, uh) to indicate interest
41. Y/N   Uses verbal summaries to confirm information
42. Y/N   Intones appropriately
43. Y/N   Reassures child
44. Y/N   Encourages child to disclose enough for further questioning
45. Y/N   Rushes child onto next phase

46. Y/N   Uses closed questions inappropriately which end
          free recall

Non-verbal aspects

47. Y/N   Child's speech fluent   50. Y/N   Interviewer's speech
                                            fluent
48. Y/N   Child is relaxed   51. Y/N   Interviewer is relaxed
49. Y/N   Child holds eye   52. Y/N   Interviewer holds eye
          contact   contact

QUESTIONING

53. Length of questioning: _____
54. Y/N   Open-ended questions asked first
55. Y/N   Specific, yet non-leading questions asked
56. Y/N   Closed questions used appropriately
57. Y/N   Leading questions used appropriately
58. Y/N   Following leading question, interviewer reverts to
          neutral questions

Interviewer:
59. Y/N   Encourages child to say s/he does not understand
60. Y/N   Uses memorable events in order to direct discussion
61. Y/N   Rephrases questions appropriately when child doesn't
          understand
62. Y/N   Picks up inconsistent statements (linguistic or factual)
63. Y/N   Asks if child has told anyone else
64. Y/N   Uses prods and continuances appropriately
65. Y/N   Discusses repeated events appropriately

OVERALL

Verbal aspects
66. Y/N   Questioning graduates from general to more specific
          information
67. Y/N   Interviewer avoids interrupting child
68. Y/N   Appropriate grammatical constructions used
69. Y/N   Double-barrelled questions used
70. Y/N   Clarification of child's terminology needed
71. Y/N   Clear account of incident obtained
72. Y/N   Questioning well structured

Non-verbal aspects

73. Y/N   Child's speech fluent

74. Y/N   Child is relaxed   79. Y/N   Interviewer is relaxed
75. Y N   Child holds eye   80. Y/N   Interviewer holds eye
      contact   contact
76. Y/N   Child is anxious   81. Y/N   Interviewer is anxious
77. Y/N   Interviewer uses   82. Y/N   Interviewer uses
      appropriate facial   appropriate body
      expressions   language
78. Y/N   Interviewer's speech
      fluent

83. Comments regarding questions asked:_____

CLOSURE

Verbal aspects

84. Y/N   Interviewer indicates termination of the interview
85. Y/N   Interviewer summarises what the witness has said
86. Y/N   Interviewer asks witness if s/he can remember anything else
87. Y/N   Interviewer uses appropriate language
88. Y/N   Interviewer assures child is not to blame
89. Y/N   Witness is given the opportunity to ask questions
90. Y/N   Witness asks questions
91. Y/N   Interviewer tells witness what will happen after the interview
92. Y/N   Interviewer thanks witness
93. Y/N   Interviewer gives child a contact name and number
94. Y/N   Interviewer explains or reiterates video-for-court issue
95. Y/N   Interviewer assesses child's competency in some way

Non-verbal aspects

96. Y/N   Witness is audible   100. Y/N   Interviewer is audible
97. Y/N   Witness' speech   101. Y/N   Interviewer's speech
      fluent   fluent
98. Y/N   Witness is relaxed   102. Y/N   Interviewer is relaxed
99. Y/N   Witness held eye   103. Y/N   Interviewer held eye
      contact   contact

Any other comments: _____

(Adapted from Wilson & Davies 1999.)

BIBLIOGRAPHY

Aldridge, M. & Wood, J. 1998, *Interviewing Children: A guide for child care and forensic practitioners*, John Wiley & Sons, Chichester.

American Psychiatric Association 1994, *Diagnostic and Statistical Manual of Mental Disorders* 4th edn, American Psychiatric Association, Washington.

Baddeley, A. 1990, *Human Memory: Theory and practice*, Lawrence Erlbaum, London.

Berliner, L. & Barbieri, M. K. 1984, 'Testimony of the child victim of sexual assault', *Journal of Social Issues*, vol. 40, pp. 125–37.

Boggs, S. & Eyberg, S. 1990, 'Interviewing techniques and establishing rapport', *Through the Eyes of the Child: Obtaining Self-Reports from Children and Adolescents*, (ed.) A. M. La Greca, Allyn and Bacon, Boston.

Bradley-Johnson, S. 1994, *Psychoeducational Assessment of Students who are Visually Impaired or Blind*, Pro-Ed, Austin.

Braithwaite, D. O. & Thompson, T. L. (eds) 2000, *Handbook of communication and people with disabilities; Research and application*, Lawrence Erlbaum Associates, Mahwah, US.

Brennan, M. & Brennan, R. E. 1990, *Strange Language: Child victims under cross examination*, 3rd edn, Riverina Literacy Centre, Wagga Wagga, NSW.

Bruck, M., Ceci, S & Francoeur, E. 2000, 'Children's use of anatomically detailed dolls to report genital touching in a medical examination: Development and gender comparisons', *Journal of Experimental Psychology: Applied*, vol. 6, pp. 74–83.

Bussey, K. 1992, 'Children's lying and truthfulness: Implications for children's testimony' in *Cognitive and Social Factors in Early Deception*, eds S. J. Ceci, M. D. Leichtman & M. E. Putnick, Lawrence Erlbaum, Hillsdale, pp. 89–109.

Butler, I. & Williamson, H. 1994, *Children Speak: Children, trauma, social work*, Longman, Harlow, Essex.

Ceci, S. J. & Bruck, M. 1993, 'The suggestibility of the child witness: A historical review and synthesis', *Psychological Bulletin*, vol. 113, pp. 403–39.

——1995, *Jeopardy in the Courtroom: A scientific analysis of children's testimony*, American Psychological Association, Washington.

Ceci, S. J., Powell, M. B. & Crossman, A. M. 1999, 'Critical issues in children's memory and testimony' in *Modern Scientific Evidence: The law and science of expert testimony*, eds D. L. Faigman, D. H. Kaye, M. J. Saks & J. Sanders, Westgroup, St Paul, pp. 40–69.

Chandler, M., Fritz, A. S. & Hala, S. 1989, 'Small-scale deceit: Deception as a marker of two-, three- and four-year-olds' early theories of mind', *Child Development*, vol. 60, no. 6, pp. 1263–77.

Clyde, J. J. 1992, The Report of the Inquiry into the Removal of Children from Orkney in February 1991, HMSO, Edinburgh.

Cole, C. B. & Loftus, E. 1987, 'The memory of children' in *Children's Eyewitness Memory*, eds S. J. Ceci, M. P. Toglia & D. F. Ross, Springer-Verlag, New York, pp. 178–208.

Davies, G., Westcott, H. & Horan, N. 2000, 'The impact of questioning style on the content of investigative interviews with suspected child sexual abuse victims', *Psychology, Crime and Law*, vol. 6, pp. 81–97.

Davies, G., Wilson, C., Mitchell, R. & Milsom, J. 1995, *Videotaping Children's Evidence: An evaluation*, Home Office, London.

DeLoache, J. S. & Marzolf, D. P. 1995, 'The use of dolls to interview young children: Issues of symbolic representation', *Journal of Experimental Child Psychology*, vol. 60, p. 155.

Fisher, R. P. 1995, 'Interviewing victims and witnesses of crime', *Psychology, Public Policy and Law*, vol. 1, pp. 732–64.

Flavell, J. H. 1985, *Cognitive Development* 2nd edn, Prentice Hall, Englewood Cliffs.

Friedman, W. 1991, 'The development of children's memory for the time of past events', *Child Development*, vol. 62, pp. 139–55.

Goodman, G. S. & Aman, C. 1990, 'Children's use of anatomically detailed dolls to recount an event', *Child Development*, vol. 61, pp. 1859–71.

Goodman, G. S., Rudy, L., Bottoms, B. L. & Aman, C. 1990, 'Children's concerns and memory: Issues of ecological validity in the study of children's eyewitness testimony' in *Knowing and Remembering in Young Children*, eds R. Fivush & J. A. Hudson, Cambridge University Press, New York, pp. 249–84.

Harnett Sheehan, K., Sheehan, D. V. & Shaw, K. R. 1988, 'Diagnosis and treatment of anxiety disorders in children and adolescents', *Psychiatric Annals*, vol. 18, pp. 146–57.

Hewitt, S. 1999, *Assessing Allegations of Sexual Abuse in Preschool Children: Understanding Small Voices*, Sage Publications, Thousand Oaks, USA.

Higgins, L. C. 1973, *Classification in the Congenitally Blind*, American Foundation for the Blind, New York.

Hudson, J. A. 1988, 'Children's memory for atypical actions in script-based stories: Evidence for a disruption effect', *Journal of Experimental Child Psychology*, vol. 46, pp. 159–73.

Hudson, J. A. & Fivush, R. 1991, 'As time goes by: Sixth graders remember a kindergarten experience', *Applied Cognitive Psychology*, vol. 5, pp. 347–60.

Hudson, J. A., Fivush, R. & Keubli, J. 1992, 'Scripts and episodes: The development of event memory', *Applied Cognitive Psychology* , vol. 6, pp. 483–505.

Hughes, M. & Grieve, R. 1980, 'On asking children bizarre questions', *First Language*, vol. 1, pp. 149–60.

Jones, D. P. H. & McGraw, J. M. 1987, 'Reliable and fictitious accounts of sexual abuse to children', *Journal of Inter-personal Violence*, vol. 2, pp. 27–45.

Katz, S., Schonfeld, D., Carter, A., Leventhal, J. & Cicchetti, D. 1995, 'The accuracy of children's reports with anatomically correct dolls', *Developmental and Behavioral Pediatrics*, vol. 16, pp. 71–6.

Kuehnle, K. 1996, *Assessing Allegations of Child Sexual Abuse*, Professional Resource Press, Miami, Florida.

Lamb, M. E., Sternberg, K. J. & Esplin, P. W. in press, 'Conducting investigative interviews of alleged sexual abuse victims', *Child Abuse and Neglect*, forthcoming.

Lamb, M. E., Sternberg, K. J., Esplin, P. W., Hershkowitz, I., Orbach, Y. & Hovav, M. 1997, 'Criterion-based content analysis: A field validation study', *Child Abuse and Neglect*, vol. 21, pp. 255–64.

Lee, H. 1960, *To Kill a Mockingbird*, Heinemann, London.

McGough, L. 1994, *Child Witnesses: Fragile voices in the American legal system*, Yale University Press, New Haven.

Milne, R. & Bull, R. 1996, 'Interviewing children with mild learning disability with the cognitive interview' in *Investigative and Forensic Decision Making*, eds N. K. Clark & G. M. Stephenson, British Psychological Society, Leicester, pp. 44–51.

Moston, S. 1987, 'The suggestibility of children in interview studies', *First Language*, vol. 7, pp. 67–78.

Murray, K. 1995, *Live Television Link: An evaluation of its use by child witnesses in Scottish criminal trials*, The Scottish Office, Edinburgh.

Nelson, K. & Gruendel, J. 1986, 'Children's scripts' in *Event Knowledge: Structure and Function in Development*, ed. K. Nelson, Lawrence Erlbaum, Hillsdale, pp. 21–47.

Peterson, C. C. 1991, 'What is a lie? Children's use of intentions and consequences in lexical definitions and moral evaluations of lying' in *Children's Interpersonal Trust*, ed. K. Rotenberg, Springer-Verlag, New York, pp. 5–19.

Peterson, C. & Biggs, M. 1997, 'Interviewing children about trauma: Problems with "specific" questions', *Journal of Traumatic Stress*, vol. 10, pp. 279–90.

Pipe, M.-E., Gee, S., Wilson, C. & Egerton, J. 1999, 'Children's recall one or two years after the event', *Developmental Psychology*, vol. 35, no. 3, pp. 781–9.

Pipe, M.-E. & Wilson, J. C. 1994, 'Cues and secrets: Influences on children's event reports', *Developmental Psychology*, vol. 30, pp. 515–25.

Ponterotto, J. G., Casas, J. M., Suzuki, L. A. & Alexander, C. M. (eds) 1995, *Handbook of Multicultural Counselling*, Sage, Thousand Oaks, pp. 181–98.

Poole, D. A. & Lamb, M. E. 1998, *Investigative Interviews of Children*, American Psychological Association, Washington.

Powell, M. B. & McMeeken, L. 1998, 'Tell me about the time when . . .': Nine golden rules for interviewing a child about a multiple offence', *Australian Police Journal*, vol. 52, no. 2, pp. 104–8.

Powell, M. B. & Thomson, D. M. 1996, 'Children's recall of an occurrence of a repeated event: Effects of age, retention interval and question type', *Child Development*, vol. 67, no. 5, pp. 1988–2004

——1997a, 'Contrasting memory for temporal source and memory for content in children's discrimination of repeated events', *Applied Cognitive Psychology*, vol. 11, pp. 339–60.

——1997b, 'The effect of intervening interview on children's ability to remember one occurrence of a repeated experience', *Legal and Criminological Psychology*, vol. 2 (part 2), pp. 247–62.

Powell, M. B., Wilson, J. C. & Croft, C. M. in press, 'The effect of uniform and prior knowledge on children's event reports and disclosure of secrets', *Police and Criminal Psychology*, forthcoming.

Prior, V., Lynch, M. & Glaser, D. 1994, *Message from Children: Children's evaluation of the professional response to child sexual abuse*, NCH Action for Children, London.

Quas, J., Qin, J., Schoaf, J. & Goodman, G. 1997, 'Individual differences in children's and adult's suggestibility and false event memory', *Learning and Individual Differences*, vol. 9, pp. 359–90.

Read, J. D. & Lindsay, D. S. 1997 *Recollections of Trauma: Scientific evidence and clinical practice*, Plenum Press, New York.

Roberts, H. & Glasgow, D. 1993, 'Gathering evidence from children: A systematic approach', *Issues in Criminological & Legal Psychology*, vol. 20, pp. 10–14.

Roberts, K. 2000, 'An overview of theory and research on children's source monitoring', *Children's Source Monitoring* (eds) K. Roberts and M. Blades, Lawrence Erlbaum, New Jersey.

Sanders, M. R. & Dadds, M. R. 1993, *Behavioral Family Intervention*, Pergamon Press, New York.

Sattler, J. M. 1998, *Clinical and Forensic Interviewing of Children and Families: Guidelines for the mental health, education, pediatric, and child maltreatment fields*, self-published, San Diego.

Saywitz, K. J. 1995, 'Improving children's testimony: The question, the answer, and the environment' in *Memory and Testimony in the Child Witness*, eds M. Zaragoza, J. Graham, G. Hall, R. Hirschman & Y. Ben-Porath, Sage, Thousand Oaks, pp. 113–40.

Seifert, K. L. & Hoffnung, R. J. 1997, *Child and Adolescent Development*, 4th edn, Houghton Mifflin Company, Boston.

Siegal, M. 1991, 'A clash of conversational worlds: Interpreting cognitive development through communication' in *Perspectives on Socially Shared Cognition*, eds L. B. Resnick, J. M. Levine & S. O. Teasley, American Psychological Association, Washington, pp. 23–40.

Spencer, J. R. & Flin, R. 1993, *The Evidence of Children: The law and the psychology*, 2nd edn, Blackstone Press, London.

Stern, W. 1939, 'The psychology of testimony', *Journal of Abnormal and Social Psychology*, vol. 34, pp. 3–20.

Sternberg, K. J., Lamb, M. E., Hershkowitz, I., Yudillevitch, L., Orbach, Y., Esplin, P. W. & Hovav, M. 1997, 'Effects of introductory style on children's abilities to describe experiences of sexual abuse', *Child Abuse and Neglect*, vol. 21, pp. 1133–46.

Stevenson, K. M , Leung, P. & Cheung, K.-F. M. 1992, 'Competency-based evaluation of interviewing skills in child sexual abuse cases', *Social Work Research and Abstracts*, vol. 28, pp. 11–16.

Thoennes, N. & Tjaden, P. 1990, 'The extent, nature and validity of sexual abuse allegations in custody visitation disputes', *Child Abuse and Neglect*, vol. 14, pp. 151–63.

Thomson, D. M. & Tulving, E. 1970, 'Associative encoding and retrieval: Weak and strong cues', *Journal of Experimental Psychology*, vol. 86, no. 2, pp. 255–62.

Vasta, R., Haith, M. M. & Miller, S. A. 1995, *Child Psychology: The modern science*, 2nd edn, John Wiley & Sons, New York.

Volbert, R. & van der Zanden, R. 1996, 'Sexual knowledge and behaviour of children up to 12 years—what is age-appropriate?' in *Psychology, Law and Criminal Justice: International developments in research and practice*, eds G. M. Davies, S. Lloyd-Bostock, M. McMurran & J. C. Wilson, de Gruyter, Berlin.

Wade, A. & Westcott, H. 1997, 'No easy answers: Child's perspectives on investigative interviews' in *Perspectives on the Memorandum: Policy, practice and research in investigative interviewing*, eds H. Westcott & J. Jones, Arena, Hants, UK.

Walker, A. G. 1994, *Handbook on Questioning Children: A linguistic perspective*, ABA Center on Children and the Law, Washington.

Walker, A. G. & Warren, A. R. 1995, 'The language of the child abuse interview: Asking the questions, understanding the answers' in *True and False Allegations of Child Sexual Abuse: Assessment and case management*, ed. T. Ney, Brunner/Mazel, New York, pp. 153–62.

Westcott, H. L. & Cross, M. 1996, *This Far and No Further: Towards ending the abuse of disabled children*, Venture Press, Birmingham.

Wilson, J. C. & Pipe, M.-E. 1995, 'The disclosure of secrets during the interviewing of children' in *Psychology and Law: Advances in research*, eds G. M. Davies, S. Lloyd-Bostock, M. McMurran & J. C. Wilson, De Gruyter, Berlin.

Wilson, J. C. & Davies, G. M. 1999, 'An evaluation of the use of videotaped evidence for juvenile witnesses in criminal courts in England and Wales', *European Journal of Criminal Policy and Research*, vol. 7, pp. 81–96.

——2000, 'An evaluation of the use of videotaped evidence interviews in child abuse investigations', *International Journal of Police Science and Management*, vol. 2, pp. 324–36.

Wood, B. S. 1981, *When the Victim is a Child: Issues for judges and prosecutors*, 2nd edn, National Institute of Justice, US Department of Justice, Washington.

Wurtele, S. K. & Miller-Perrin, C. L. 1992, *Preventing Child Sexual Abuse: Sharing the responsibility*, University of Nebraska Press, Lincoln.

Yuille, J. C. 1991, 'The Step-wise Interview: A protocol for interviewing children', unpublished manuscript, University of British Columbia.

INDEX